Practical Resuscitation

D0805146

Dedications

To our families for their unyielding love and support and to those personally and professionally known, who have inspired our passion to improve recognition of and response to resuscitation emergencies.

Practical Resuscitation:

Recognition
and
Response

EDITED BY

Pam Moule
RN, DipN, DipNE, BSc (Hons), MSc
Principal Lecturer
University of the West of England,
Bristol

AND

John W Albarran
RN, Dip N (Lon.), BSc (Hons), PG Dip Ed, MSc,
NFESC
Principal Lecturer
University of the West of England,
Bristol

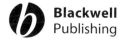
Blackwell Publishing

© 2005 by Blackwell Publishing Ltd

Editorial offices:
Blackwell Publishing Ltd, 9600 Garsington Road, Oxford OX4 2DQ, UK
    Tel: +44 (0)1865 776868
Blackwell Publishing Inc., 350 Main Street, Malden, MA 02148-5020, USA
    Tel: +1 781 388 8250
Blackwell Publishing Asia Pty Ltd, 550 Swanston Street, Carlton, Victoria
3053, Australia
    Tel: +61 (0)3 8359 1011

The right of the Authors to be identified as the Authors of this Work has
been asserted in accordance with the Copyright, Designs and Patents Act
1988.

First published 2005 by Blackwell Publishing Ltd

Library of Congress Cataloging-in-Publication Data
Practical resuscitation: recognition and response / edited by Pam Moule
and John W. Albarran.
        p. ; cm.
    Includes bibliographical references and index.
    ISBN 1-4051-1668-4 (pbk. : alk. paper)
    1. Resuscitation.   2. Emergency nursing.
    [DNLM: 1. Resuscitation–methods.   2. Emergency
    Treatment–methods.   WA 292 P896 2005]   I. Moule, Pam.
    II. Albarran, John W.

    RC87.9.P73 2005
    616.02′5–dc22

                                                    2004014741

ISBN-10 1-4051-1668-4
ISBN-13 978 14051 1668 8

A catalogue record for this title is available from the British Library

Set in 9 on 11pt Palatino
by SNP Best-set Typesetter Ltd., Hong Kong
Printed and bound in India
by Replika Press Pvt, Ltd, Kundli

For further information on Blackwell Publishing, visit our website:
www.blackwellnursing.com

Contents

Foreword

There are few greater challenges to the skills and ability of a healthcare provider than those posed by the patient in cardiac arrest. In no other condition do the actions of those who first manage the patient have such a profound influence on survival. Many who provide the initial care for such patients are relatively junior with limited experience, but their actions may literally mean the difference between life and death.

The skills required during a resuscitation attempt are essentially practical, although underpinned by sound theoretical principles. In this book *Practical Resuscitation: recognition and response*, several experts have collaborated to provide a very readable approach to the acquisition of both the theoretical knowledge required and the practical techniques needed to resuscitate the victim of cardiopulmonary arrest. The approach in all cases is practical, depending on skills in assessment of the casualty, with subsequent actions determined by the findings. The rationale behind these actions is explained, as are the techniques required. Finally, the practitioner is encouraged to reflect on the events that have taken place and use this process to learn and improve further.

After sections on ethical and professional issues, the basic principles of resuscitation medicine and the equipment used are described. Chapters then progress logically from basic life support to advanced techniques, with several chapters devoted to more specialised aspects of advanced life support. The overall result is a comprehensive introduction that will serve the newcomer to the hospital ward well, as well as the more experienced practitioner undertaking an extended role. While intended primarily for nurses, it is equally suitable for medical or paramedical staff who may participate in resuscitation attempts or who wish to learn more about the subject.

All the authors are based in the west of England, in Gloucester or Bristol, and are to be congratulated for producing an eminently readable account that is both a practical introduction to the subject as well as a manual for learning and applying practical skills in the treatment of patients. At the same time it provides a comprehensive introduction at a more advanced level, to a subject of increasing importance in modern healthcare. In no small way is this also due to the skilful editorship of Pam Moule and John Albarran, two stalwarts of nurse education, based at the University of the West of England.

With the skills that can be learnt from this volume, the basis of sound practice will be established and serve the reader well in practice whether working as a first responder, a member of the cardiac arrest team or as the team leader.

Michael Colquhoun
Chairman, Resuscitation Council (UK)
Wales College of Medicine
University of Cardiff
Cardiff

Preface

The field of resuscitation is an area where theory and practice are developing at a very rapid pace. Advances in technology and an increase in the number of published quality research papers mean that guidelines are revised periodically so that standards in cardiopulmonary resuscitation can reflect the most current thinking and application of technical skills. The increased patient dependency, now common within many hospital and community settings, has further emphasised the need for healthcare professionals to become competent in basic life support and, increasingly, immediate life support skills.

The premise behind this book is that healthcare professionals starting their career as practitioners need to be equipped with a blend of theoretical and practice-based skills in order to be effective as first responders, resuscitation team members or leaders of the arrest situation. This textbook therefore approaches knowledge and skill development in resuscitation from a practical viewpoint and introduces the concept of the '3Rs', namely *recognition*, *response* and *review*.

To this end, we have adopted the idea of 'recognition' as a process that involves assessing the patient and determining whether the individual is unconscious or suffering a cardiac arrest. Within this phase other clinical features and patient data must be considered before 'responding'. Included here is the idea of taking action based on the cause of the arrest. This requires decision and action. Through this format we hope to have developed an accessible text for the novice. The final R relates to 'reviewing' actions and decisions taken or omitted but this can also be interpreted as reviewing what has been learned.

There is no doubt that the first experience of participating in an arrest is terrifying, whatever the role or activity adopted. We expect the reader will become more confident and proficient in recognising, responding to and reviewing resuscitation situations. Moreover, we hope that this text will stimulate greater interest and enthusiasm in the resuscitation field.

Pam Moule and John W Albarran

Acknowledgements

The editors are grateful to the following staff from the University of the West of England, Bristol:

- Adrian Guy, Audio Visual Technician; Dave Watkins, Senior Skills Technician; and Neil Wakeman, Skills Technician, for their assistance with photographs;
- Jane Wathen, Graphic Designer, for help with some of the images;
- Philip Tubman, On-line Learning Designer, for help with composing some of the images;
- To a number of colleagues who kindly gave their time and agreed to pose for the photographs in this textbook.

We also owe thanks to:

- Gloucestershire Hospitals NHS Trust for permission to reproduce their charts in Chapter 2;
- Blackwell Publishing, for permission to use published material from Jevon (2003) in Chapter 2;
- Resuscitation Council UK for permission to use algorithms in a number of chapters.

Contributors

John W Albarran
(Chapters 8 & 9)

Principal Lecturer
University of the West of England
Bristol

Rebecca Hoskins
(Chapter 11)

Nurse Consultant in Emergency Care
United Bristol Hospitals Trust and
University of the West of England
Bristol

Ben King
(Chapters 4, 12 & 15)

Senior Resuscitation Officer
Gloucestershire Royal Hospital
Gloucester

Una McKay
(Chapters 3 & 7)

Clinical Skills Demonstrator, ALS Trainer
University of the West of England
Bristol

Pam Moule
(Chapters 5 & 9)

Principal Lecturer
University of the West of England
Bristol

Paul Snelling
(Chapters 1, 2 & 10)

Senior Lecturer
University of the West of England
Gloucestershire

Dr Jas Soar
(Chapter 14)

Consultant in Anaesthesia and Intensive
   Care Medicine
Southmead Hospital
Bristol

Jackie Younker
(Chapters 6, 7 & 13)

Senior Lecturer
University of the West of England
Bristol

How to Use the Book

STRUCTURE AND CONTENT

The book is divided into five sections, which aim to offer a comprehensive insight into current concepts.

(1) Professional issues – reviews professional, legal and ethical issues and discusses the role of the healthcare worker in resuscitation.
(2) Prevention and preparation – recognising the sick patient, preventing cardiac arrest and resuscitation equipment are discussed.
(3) Basic life support – provides an overview of the Chain of Survival and basic life support algorithm.
(4) Advanced life support – reviews the advanced life support algorithm and considers associated knowledge and skills, including post-resuscitation care.
(5) Further considerations of resuscitation – reviews the delivery of resuscitation in a number of special circumstances, including resuscitation of the infant and child.

Each section contains chapters written by experts in their area, that inform and develop through the provision of evidence-based guidance. Every chapter is presented in an accessible manner, using a structure that includes the following elements.

- Introduction – an overview of the chapter content.
- Aims – guide the reader to the key aims of the chapter, enabling selective and appropriate reading.
- Learning outcomes – identify the key learning for the reader.
- Content (guidelines, evidence-based literature, steps in the skill) – provides the reader with the knowledge development and evidence base, stressing practice skill delivery.
- Review of learning – provides a useful and concise resumé of key learning for the reader.

- Case studies – offer an opportunity for readers to test their understanding and development of the key issues presented in the chapter.
- Reference list – provides the reader with an opportunity to further explore reference material and develop wider reading.

PRACTICAL USE

The evidence base presented will support care delivery, whilst key skill delivery, presented through a step-by-step approach, should enhance confidence and competence development. Summary boxes reflecting the key learning within chapters afford an opportunity to review individual learning.

The case study examples provide scope to test individual understanding of the evidence base and steps in skill delivery, which can be further enhanced through exploration of the reference material provided within each chapter.

Section 1

Introduction and Professional Issues

1 | Professional, Ethical and Legal Issues

INTRODUCTION
International collaboration has supported the development of resuscitation guidelines that seek to provide a consensus view for practice. This chapter outlines major ethical, professional and legal issues surrounding resuscitation and presents roles and responsibilities of the 'first responder' in an emergency arrest situation.

AIMS
This chapter introduces professional issues in resuscitation and gives an overview of the roles of healthcare professionals in a resuscitation attempt.

LEARNING OUTCOMES
By the end of the chapter the reader will be able to:

❑ discuss the ethical and legal implications of *do not attempt resuscitation' orders*;
❑ explore the debates related to the *presence of family members* during resuscitation;
❑ examine the ethical dilemmas associated with deciding *when to discontinue resuscitation attempts*;
❑ appreciate the *different roles of cardiac arrest team members* and how to work with the team.

'DO NOT ATTEMPT RESUSCITATION' ORDERS
Joint guidance from the British Medical Association, the Royal College of Nursing and the Resuscitation Council UK (2001) forms the basis for the 'do not attempt resuscitation' (DNAR) policy.

The wishes of the patient

It is firmly established in law and ethics that a competent patient can refuse any treatment whatever, for any reason (Mason & McCall Smith 1999) and any health professional who disregards these wishes is vulnerable to legal challenge. A more difficult situation is where a competent patient requests that resuscitation attempts be made where there is no hope for success and the healthcare team do not believe that it is indicated. The doctor cannot be *required* to undertake any procedure, including resuscitation, which is not clinically indicated.

Ascertaining the patient's wishes

Good practice (Resuscitation Council UK 2001) requires that the issue of resuscitation is explored in a sensitive way. In one study, 86% of elderly patients stated that they were willing to be consulted about their resuscitation status (Mead & Turnbull 1995). However, more recent evidence suggests that involving patients in such crucial decisions is not always performed (Costello 2002). However, information and discussion should not be forced on individuals who do not wish it.

Advance directives

Advance directives or 'living wills' are statements made by competent patients, giving details of their wishes about future treatment options. Though there is no legislation covering their use, they are legally binding in certain circumstances. To be valid the patient should:

- intend the advance directive to apply in the circumstances;
- be mentally competent when the advance directive was made;
- not have been influenced by another person;
- be aware of the risks and complications of the treatments (Resuscitation Council UK 2000a).

Decision making in the case of patients deemed incompetent

Where patients lack the capacity to make an informed decision, the duty for making a decision in the patient's best interest falls not to the family but to the medical team. There is an assumption that people are competent to make their own decisions (Nursing and Midwifery Council 2002). Where there is doubt, the test, based on the legal case of *Re: C* (1994), is that the patient should:

- comprehend and retain treatment information;
- believe it;
- be able to weigh it in the balance and make a choice (McHale 2002).

If there is serious dispute about the decision, a second opinion can be sought from other clinicians. Rarely, a legal opinion may be requested (Pennels 2001).

The outcome of the resuscitation attempt

The joint guidance (Resuscitation Council UK 2001) gives three examples of where resuscitation can be withheld on grounds of suspected poor outcome.

- Where attempting cardiopulmonary resuscitation (CPR) will not restart the patient's heart and breathing.
- Where there is no benefit in restarting the patient's heart.
- Where the expected benefit is outweighed by the projected burdens.

Making and communicating the decision

When a decision has been made, it is vitally important that it is communicated to all in the healthcare team in the following ways.

- The entry in the medical notes should be clear and unambiguous, with no use of abbreviations.
- The date and the reason for the decision should be clear.
- There should be details of who has been consulted.
- The signature should be easily identifiable.
- A separate entry should also be made in the nursing notes.
- The decision should be reviewed regularly and can be rescinded at any time (Resuscitation Council UK 2001).

WHEN TO STOP A RESUSCITATION ATTEMPT
The decision making will depend on a number of factors.

- The environment of the cardiac arrest and access to emergency medical services.
- The interval between cardiac arrest and commencement of basic life support (BLS).
- The interval between BLS and advanced life support (ALS).
- Evidence of cardiac death (asystole).
- Potential prognosis and co-morbidity (Ambery *et al.* 2000).
- Age of the casualty, but this is a controversial issue (Larkin 2002).
- Temperature: hypothermia offers a degree of protection and efforts, prolonged if necessary, should be made to warm the patient (see Chapter 11).
- Drug intake prior to cardiac arrest.
- Remediable precipitating factors (Resuscitation Council UK 2000a).

Resuscitation should continue if there is any evidence of cardiac electrical activity and should only cease if asystole is present. It has been recommended that patients should be monitored for ten minutes after resuscitation efforts have stopped (Maleck *et al.* 1998). The final decision rests with the team leader, though it should be made in consultation with the cardiac arrest team (Gabbott *et al.* 2000).

HAVING FAMILY MEMBERS PRESENT DURING CARDIOPULMONARY RESUSCITATION
Reasons for allowing family members to attend the resuscitation of a relative include the following:

- family-centred care movement (e.g. hospice movement and in paediatric nursing);
- public demand for greater openness and transparency;
- research evidence.

One of the major driving forces for change relates to the pioneering work of the Foote Hospital, Michigan (Doyle *et al.* 1987). In this study only 47 questionnaires were returned complete; of these, 76% (*n* = 36) of the respondents stated that their adjustment to the patient's death was made easier by being present; 64% ($n = 30$) believed their presence was beneficial to the patient and 94% ($n = 44$) indicated that they would attend again.

The Resuscitation Council UK (1996) and the American Heart Association, in collaboration with the International Liaison Committee on Resuscitation (2000), have issued guidelines supporting the concept of family presence but despite this, there is still resistance to change practice (Newton 2002).

Excluding family members

Although there are many reasons cited for excluding family members from the resuscitation of a patient, most are based on speculation and paternalistic attitudes rather than evidence from research (Albarran & Stafford 1999).

- Family members will physically interfere with treatments and require restraining.
- The incidence of legal actions taken against healthcare professionals will increase.
- Allowing family members to witness the resuscitation is a breach of the patient's confidentiality.
- The presence of family members will affect staff performance.
- The psychological consequences of family presence during CPR are unknown.
- There is insufficient evidence to endorse wholesale change in practice.
- Conflicting attitudes of nursing and medical staff.

Arguments in favour of family members being allowed into the resuscitation room

Even when resuscitation attempts have been unsuccessful, family members are able to describe a number of benefits.

- Family members can witness the efforts of the resuscitation team which may dispel any doubts about how the patient died.
- Attendance can demystify the process of CPR, reduce misconceptions and prevent family members creating distorted images of the procedures involved.

- Relatives are able to touch, stroke and kiss the patient while their body is still warm.
- Family members have the opportunity to express their feelings of love, encouragement or whatever as there might be a faint chance that the patient will hear and/or be reassured that their loved ones are at the bedside.
- Family members gain a sense that they have a role in supporting the patient.
- Family members humanise the situation and the patient is viewed in a social context.
- Being present in the final moments is comforting for many relatives, promotes closure and enables them to start to grieve.
- Early psychological adjustment and reduced emotional distress may result if family members attend the resuscitation of a loved one.
- Closer relationships can be formed between the clinical staff and patient's family (Williams 2002).

Supporting the family member during resuscitation of a relative

Having a hospital-wide policy is vital for directing healthcare staff in managing such situations. In deciding whether family members should be invited to witness CPR of a relative, the following issues should be considered (Albarran & Stafford 1999).

- The nature of the request.
- Appropriateness of the situation.
- Staffing. An experienced individual must be assigned to escort and remain with the relatives and act as interpreter for interventions and procedures being undertaken.
- Team decision. All members of the resuscitation team should be in agreement.
- Timing. Ideally this should be during less invasive procedures and when the patient is not soaked in blood or other bodily fluids.
- Physical and emotional harm. Fulbrook (1998) has raised concerns that the risk of litigation is more likely if a relative

suffers harm during their experience as a witness. Staff must also explain procedures such as defibrillation and the principles behind resuscitation.

Finally, it is also essential that there are facilities for staff to debrief and to receive counselling.

OFF-DUTY STAFF

In most situations there is a clear moral duty for healthcare staff to attend a casualty when not at work but at present there is no legal requirement to do so in the UK. There is clear guidance in the new *Code of Professional Conduct* (Nursing and Midwifery Council 2002) regarding a professional duty to offer emergency assistance.

There is some concern that legal action may be brought as a result of a resuscitation attempt in the community (Resuscitation Council UK 2000b). The paucity of cases in this area makes it difficult to come to any definite conclusions but health professionals are advised:

- to follow guidelines recommended by authoritative bodies;
- to check the extent of personal indemnity insurance.

A discussion paper with further advice is available from the Resuscitation Council UK (2000b): www.resus.org.uk/pages/legal.htm.

ROLE OF THE HEALTHCARE PROFESSIONAL AT RESUSCITATION

The initial management sequence

A respiratory or cardiac arrest may occur at any time and any place within the healthcare environment. Though these may be unproblematic, complications can exist, such as the patient who is:

- in a wheelchair with a bilateral amputation of their legs;
- prone on the operating table mid procedure;
- collapsed whilst on the toilet and has become wedged between the toilet and the cubicle wall;

- in the bath;
- on the treadmill during an exercise test in the cardiology department;
- found hanging from the fire escape following a suicide attempt.

Or it may be a member of staff who has arrested in the hospital canteen.

In responding to any situation it is imperative that first responders ensure their own safety. Only then can they begin to deal with the situation.

The following issues need to be considered.

Assessment of the patient

Assess the patient in the position in which you find them for responsiveness, breathing and circulation. Ensure that the patient is for active resuscitation and does not have a 'do not attempt resuscitation' (DNAR) order placed on them.

Call for appropriate help

Activate any emergency buzzer in the department to ensure a quick response from your colleagues. Generally, there will always be other staff members around, allowing one or two people to deal with the patient whilst other members of the team dial the cardiac arrest number and fetch the emergency equipment to the patient. The person who makes the call for the cardiac arrest team should ensure that they dial the correct number. It is important to be clear and calm when talking to the operator. All staff should also be aware of where the nearest cardiac arrest trolley and defibrillator are located.

Get the patient into a supine position suitable for resuscitation to commence. If the patient is in bed, it is not absolutely essential for the headboard to be removed before airway management may commence.

Ensure that the mattress type is suitable for performing resuscitation. There are some mattresses that are unsuitable when chest compressions are being performed on a patient, such as an air mattress that will need to be deflated in the appropriate manner.

Arrested patient

Two-person basic resuscitation should commence and the arrival of the cardiac arrest team should be anticipated, as highlighted in Chapter 5. Remember that by the time the team arrives, the following should be occurring.

- Airway management being performed with either a pocket mask or bag-valve-mask, ideally with oxygen attached.
- Chest compressions being performed at the appropriate rate and depth and in co-ordination with airway management.
- Reasonable space around the patient to allow safe working of the team.
- Cardiac arrest equipment at the patient's bedside, particularly the defibrillator, which may already have been used if staff are appropriately trained.
- Cardiac monitoring has been established.
- Intravenous access may have been established or any existing access confirmed to be in working order.
- The patient's notes and drug chart immediately available.

The cardiac arrest team members and how to work with them

Most cardiac arrest teams will consist of the following healthcare workers.

- Medical senior house officer (SHO) and/or registrar (generally assume team leader role)
- Medical house officer (HO)
- Anaesthetist (and often an assistant such as an operating department practitioner/assistant (ODP/ODA) or intensive care/anaesthetic nurse)
- Senior nurse (may be departmental senior nurse or clinical site manager)
- Resuscitation officer (RO)

In addition to the team, there are likely to be several staff members from the ward or department who will stay with the patient and work with the team. These members are important, as often they will have the best knowledge of the patient.

To ensure a co-ordinated approach, the Resuscitation Council UK (2000a) suggests that the cardiac arrest team meets daily, preferably at the beginning of any new shift, and appoints a team leader in the event of a cardiac arrest call.

The following healthcare professionals perform essential skills.

- *Medical registrar* – acting as cardiac arrest team leader, standing back from the patient to achieve a good overview of the activities of the team and give clear directions accordingly.
- *Medical house officer* – attempting to achieve intravenous access so that drugs can be administered quickly.
- *Anaesthetist* – managing the airway with bag-valve-mask ventilation.
- *Intensive care nurse* – assisting the anaesthetist.
- *Student nurse* – performing chest compressions under the supervision and support of the intensive care nurse.
- *Ward sister* – performing defibrillation.

The Resuscitation Council UK (2003) gives very clear guidance on the role of the cardiac arrest team leader and the individual team members.

POST ARREST

Following any resuscitation attempt, successful or not, a number of tasks will need to be undertaken. These are considered in detail in Chapter 12 and will include:

- completion of the cardiac arrest audit or report form;
- restocking the cardiac arrest trolley;
- dealing with relatives;
- debriefing for the cardiac arrest team.

REVIEW OF LEARNING

- ❏ Resuscitation is not always appropriate in persons who suffer cardiac arrest.
- ❏ Patients' wishes on their resuscitation status should usually be sought and respected.
- ❏ Family members should be allowed to witness resuscitation attempts provided certain conditions are met.

❏ There is a professional duty for healthcare professionals to offer emergency treatment.
❏ Good assessment and consideration of the environment are essential in the initial management of the arrested patient.
❏ Resuscitation may be attempted prior to the arrival of the team, then continue with effective team working.
❏ Following resuscitation, a number of tasks need completing such as debriefing and audit form completion.

CONCLUSION

This chapter considers the introduction to resuscitation, reviewing professional issues and roles at resuscitation events. The remaining chapters support the development of clinical competence through presenting a comprehensive evidence base in resuscitation: recognition and response.

REFERENCES

Albarran, J.W. & Stafford, H. (1999) Resuscitation and family presence: implications for nurses in critical areas. *Advancing Clinical Nursing* **3** (1), 11–19.

Ambery, P., King, B. & Banerjee, M. (2000) Does concurrent or previous illness accurately predict cardiac arrest survival? *Resuscitation* **47**, 267–71.

American Heart Association/International Liaison Committee on Resuscitation (2000) Guidelines for cardiopulmonary resuscitation and emergency cardiovascular care. *Circulation* **102** (suppl 8), 1–374.

Costello, J. (2002) Do Not Resuscitate orders and older patients: findings from an ethnographic study of hospital wards for older people. *Journal of Advanced Nursing* **39** (5), 491–9.

Doyle, C.J., Post, H., Maino, J., Keefe, M. & Rhee, K. (1987) Family participation during resuscitation: an option. *Annals of Emergency Medicine* **16** (6), 673–5.

Fulbrook, S. (1998) Medico-legal insights: legal implications of relatives witnessing resuscitation. *British Journal of Theatre Nursing* **7** (10), 33–5.

Gabbott, D., Walmsley, H. & Pateman, J. (2000) *Guidance for Clinical Practice and Training in Hospitals*. Resuscitation Council UK, London. Available online at: www.resus.org.uk/pages/standard.htm

Larkin, G.L. (2002) Termination of resuscitation: the art of clinical decision making. *Current Opinion in Critical Care* **8** (3), 224–9.

Maleck, W.H., Piper, S.N., Triem, J., Boldt, J. & Zittel, F.U. (1998) Unexpected return of spontaneous circulation after cessation of resuscitation (Lazarus phenomenon). *Resuscitation* **39**, 125–8.

Mason, J.K. & McCall Smith, R.A. (1999) *Law and Medical Ethics*, 5th edn. Butterworths, London.

McHale, J. (2002) Consent and the capable adult patient. In: Tingle, J. & Cribb, A. (eds) (2002) *Nursing Law and Ethics*, 2nd edn. Blackwell Publishing, London.

Mead, G.E. & Turnbull, C.J. (1995) Cardiopulmonary resuscitation in the elderly: patients' and relatives' views. *Journal of Medical Ethics* **21** (1), 39–44.

Newton, A. (2002) Witnessed resuscitation in critical care: the case against. *Intensive and Critical Care Nursing* **18**, 146–50.

Nursing and Midwifery Council (2002) *Code of Professional Conduct*. Nursing and Midwifery Council, London.

Pennels, C. (2001) Resuscitation: the legal and ethical implications. *Professional Nurse* **16** (11), 1476–7.

Re C (Adult: Refusal of Medical Treatment) [1994] 1 All ER 819, [1994] 1 WLR 290.

Resuscitation Council UK (1996) *Should Relatives Witness Resuscitation?* A report from a project team of the Resuscitation Council UK. Resuscitation Council UK, London.

Resuscitation Council UK (2000a) *Advanced Life Support Course Provider Manual*, 4th edn. Resuscitation Council UK, London.

Resuscitation Council UK (2000b) *The Legal Status of Those Who Attempt Resuscitation.* Resuscitation Council UK, London. Available online at: www.resus.org.uk/pages/legal.htm

Resuscitation Council UK (2001) *Decisions Relating to Cardiopulmonary Resuscitation*. A joint statement from the British Medical Association, the Resuscitation Council UK and the Royal College of Nursing. Available online at: www.resus.org/pages/dnar.htm

Resuscitation Council UK (2003) *Advanced Life Support Course Provider Manual Appendix, The Cardiac Arrest Team Leader and Team*, 4th edn. Resuscitation Council UK, London.

Williams, J.M. (2002) Family presence during resuscitation: to see or not see? *Nursing Clinics of North America* **37** (1), 211–20.

Section 2

Prevention and Preparation

2 Recognising the Sick Patient and Preventing Cardiac Arrest

INTRODUCTION

Despite its popular portrayal, cardiorespiratory arrest is often neither sudden nor unpredictable (Resuscitation Council UK 2000). Studies over several years have shown that most cardiac arrests are avoidable if signs and symptoms are recognised and responded to (Franklin & Mathew 1994, Hodgetts *et al.* 2002a, Smith & Wood 1998). Patients with coronary artery disease are more likely to have a sudden cardiac arrest, often precipitated by an unstable area of ischaemic myocardium. Such events will be heralded by the onset of symptoms in many cases. At least 80% of individuals who suffer sudden cardiac death have coronary artery disease (Zipes & Wellens 1998) and so any strategy to prevent cardiac arrest must begin here. Recognising and responding to patients at risk of deterioration and cardiac arrest is a clinical priority.

AIMS

This chapter introduces the principles of prevention of cardiac arrest by:

- understanding how to recognise and respond to acute coronary syndromes;
- understanding how to recognise life-threatening deterioration using structured assessment;
- discussing methods of obtaining rapid medical advice and intervention for patients whose condition is deteriorating.

LEARNING OUTCOMES

At the end of the chapter the reader should be able to:

- ❏ identify the *classification and pathophysiology* of acute coronary syndrome;

❏ discuss the *diagnosis and treatments* for acute coronary syndrome;

❏ describe how deteriorating patients should be *assessed using a systematic approach*;

❏ identify the importance of *calling for expert help rapidly*;

❏ discuss ways of *triggering assistance*.

ACUTE CORONARY SYNDROME

Nearly a quarter of a million people each year in England and Wales suffer from an acute myocardial infarction (AMI) (Gerschlick 2001). Up to half of these will die within a month and over half of these deaths occur before the patient reaches hospital (NICE 2002a), many within the first few minutes of the onset of symptoms (DoH 2000a). It is well known that the chance of survival following an AMI is dramatically increased if treatment is initiated early. It is vital therefore that AMI is recognised promptly and treatment initiated immediately. This applies equally to patients who suffer AMI out of hospital and those who are already hospital inpatients.

The term 'acute coronary syndrome' (ACS) has recently become popular to describe the three main clinical presentations of unstable coronary artery disease (Jones 2003). They are:

- unstable angina
- non-ST elevation myocardial infarction (NSTEMI)
- ST elevation myocardial infarction (STEMI).

Pathophysiology

The vast majority of ACS is caused by thrombosis developing at the site of an atherosclerotic plaque in a coronary artery (Davies 2000). As the plaque grows, it gradually occludes the lumen of the artery, thus reducing the amount of blood flow. Plaques are composed of a lipid core covered by a fibrous cap (Jowett & Thompson 2003) (see Figure 2.1).

ACS is most frequently caused by the development of a blood clot at the site of the plaque. Usually this occurs where the outer covering of the plaque ruptures, exposing the thrombogenic inner core to blood in the arterial lumen (Davies 2000). Platelet aggregation and fibrin deposition occur (Jowett & Thompson

2003). Initially the thrombus forms in the plaque and then extends into the lumen.

The presentations of ACS are caused in slightly different ways.

- If the clot partially occludes the lumen, resulting in sharply reduced blood flow, unstable angina results.
- If the clot occludes the lumen but spontaneously dissolves or if there is distal embolisation causing myocardial damage, NSTEMI results.
- If the clot completely occludes the lumen, AMI involving the full thickness of the ventricular wall will result. This is associated with ST segment elevation on the electrocardiogram (ECG). In this case a STEMI has occurred.

Figure 2.2 shows how the pathophysiology and ECG changes are linked. The diagnosis and therefore treatment of ACS in the acute phase are based on clinical history, evidence of risk factors and the ECG changes rather than the pathological processes described above. It is recognised that there is a continuum between unstable angina and NSTEMI (British Cardiac Society 2001).

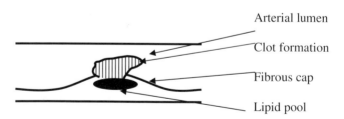

Fig. 2.1 Clot formation at the site of an atheromatous plaque.

Condition	Pathophysiology	Typical ECG trace*	Biochemical markers
Stable angina	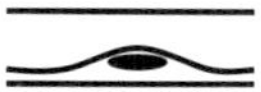 Stable plaque	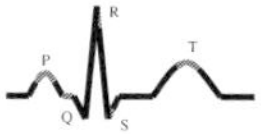 Can be normal	Absent
Unstable angina	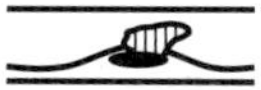 Clot formation	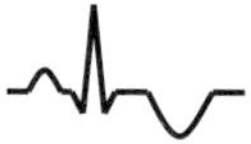 T wave inversion	Absent
NSTEMI	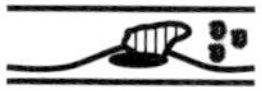 Distal embolisation	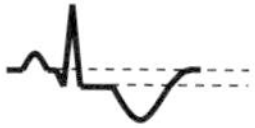 ST segment depression	Present
STEMI	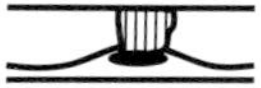 Full artery occlusion	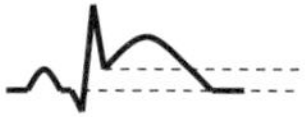 ST segment elevation	Present

* These are typical ECG presentations – different ECG morphology or normal ECG is possible

Fig. 2.2 Classification in acute coronary syndrome.

Clinical presentation

- Pain. This is the initial response to myocardial ischaemia. Typically the pain is central and gripping in nature. Commonly it radiates to the left arm, though pain can be reported anywhere in the chest, arms, neck, jaw and teeth (Albarran 2002). However, up to 25% of AMIs are 'silent' (pain free), more commonly in people aged over 65 and diabetics (Hand 2001).
- Nausea and vomiting.
- Hypotension.
- Anxiety.
- Tachycardia.
- Pale, clammy skin.

Chest pain or any other suspected ACS should be treated as a medical emergency. Up to 30% of patients with acute chest pain are suffering from ACS (Domanovits et al. 2002). At presentation the goals are:

- relief of symptoms;
- diagnosis, including investigations;
- specific treatment.

Relief of symptoms

These are often categorised by the mnemonic MONA (Resuscitation Council UK 2000).

M Morphine (or diamorphine). This should be given intravenously (IV). Cannulation is a priority. Intravenous antiemetic (e.g. metoclopramide 10 mg) is often given at the same time. Intramuscular injections should be avoided.

O Oxygen, in a high concentration.

N Nitroglycerine (GTN) spray, to dilate the coronary arteries.

A Aspirin 300 mg orally.

Diagnosis

Diagnosis is by history, assessment of risk factors, clinical examination and thorough investigations. The commonest and most important investigation is the electrocardiogram (ECG).

This should be performed as soon as possible, as treatment decisions are heavily influenced by it.

Electrocardiogram

Electrocardiographic changes can be detected after only 30–60 seconds of ischaemia (Edwards 2002), although they may develop later or return back to baseline (Albarran & Kapeluch 2000). Strips from a cardiac monitor should not be used to diagnose ACS; each lead of the ECG shows a different area of the heart and any lead not recording an area of damage may appear perfectly normal. A full 12-lead ECG, repeated frequently, is required. Regions of damage in the heart are identified by characteristic patterns in ECG leads. Readers are referred to more specialised books for further details (see Jevon 2003). All clinical areas should have access to a 12-lead ECG machine 24 hours a day and where an area does not possess such facilities, arrangements for rapid access should be in place.

Any changes in an ECG must be interpreted in the light of the history and condition of the patient. A normal ECG does not exclude AMI and some 'abnormalities' can occur normally. If symptoms are sufficiently serious to warrant an ECG, then they are also sufficiently serious for it to be interpreted immediately. The changes in ECG morphology most associated with ACS are given in Figure 2.2. Figure 2.3 depicts a 12-lead ECG showing the characteristic ST elevation in the leads looking at the inferior surface of the heart.

Biochemical markers

When cardiac cells are damaged, intracellular proteins leak out and can be detected in the blood. The most important and accurate of these are the cardiac troponins (Harrison 1999). Troponins are also useful for assessing the risk of further events (Galvani *et al.* 1997). Other markers are:

- creatine phosphokinase (CK);
- lactate dehydrogenase (LDH);
- serum glutamic oxaloacetic transaminase (SGOT) (Jowett & Thompson 2003).

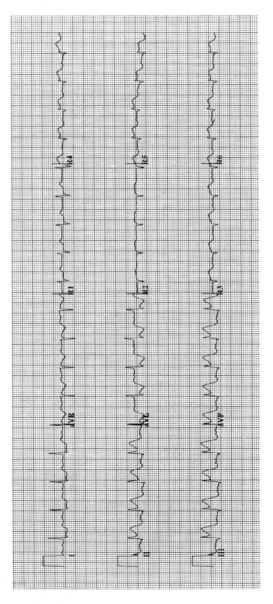

Fig. 2.3 Acute inferior myocardial infarction (from Jevon (2003) with permission from Blackwell Publishing).

These markers are useful in diagnosis, although elevation of CK (CK-MB) is more specific to cardiac necrosis rather than other muscle damage (Jowett & Thompson 2003). However, as the levels of some enzymes do not start to rise until 2–8 hours after injury, their role in the diagnosis of ACS is limited. Since these enzymes are not present solely in cardiac cells, elevated levels could be due to a number of causes, including intramuscular injection. Blood samples are needed to complete serial measurement of biochemical markers, though the exact tests performed will vary between hospitals. Measurement by these enzymes, though performed in most hospitals (Baron *et al.* 2004), has been superseded by cardiac troponins, which are far superior in terms of sensitivity and specificity. Moreover, raised levels can be detected earlier and are also of value in classifying patients into ACS subgroups.

TREATMENT

Non-ST elevation myocardial infarction and unstable angina

The treatment for these two conditions can be considered together. Anticoagulant and antiplatelet therapy can prevent progression to STEMI (Hughes 2003) by limiting expansion of the thrombus so that it does not completely occlude the vessel. Treatment with thrombolytic drugs should not be given (Jowett & Thompson 2003).

- Heparin, either as infusion or low molecular weight given subcutaneously, reduces risk.
- In high-risk patients an infusion of a glycoprotein IIa/IIIb inhibitor can be considered (Stevens 2002). These drugs (abciximab, eptifibatide and tirofiban) inhibit platelet aggregation and are given as infusions with heparin and aspirin (NICE 2002b).

ST elevation myocardial infarction

Once ST elevation myocardial infarction has been diagnosed, and if there are no contraindications (see Table 2.1), thrombolysis should be commenced immediately. Thrombolytic drugs dissolve the blood clot, re-establishing blood flow to the ischaemic myocardium. Timing of administration is vitally important and treatment should be given as soon as possible (normally up to 12 hours) after the onset of chest pain (Albarran & Kapeluch 2000). Many hospitals have care pathways for AMI and protocols that detail drug administration. The four drugs currently available (NICE 2002a) are:

- streptokinase – this is the oldest and cheapest drug. Because antibodies are produced after its administration it can only be given once. It is given as an IV infusion over 1 hour;
- alteplase – this can be given in two different ways, both involving bolus injections and infusions;
- reteplase – this is given as two IV injections 30 minutes apart;
- tenecteplase – this can be given as a single IV injection and so is suitable for out-of-hospital administration.

Streptokinase costs less than £100 per person, while the other three cost £600–800 per person (NICE 2002a). Perhaps for this reason, streptokinase is at present the most widely used. A heparin infusion is given with alteplase, reteplase and tenecteplase.

Table 2.1 Cautions and contraindications of thrombolysis (BNF 2003).

Cautions	Contraindications
Bleeding from recent invasive procedures	Recent haemorrhage, trauma or surgery
External chest compressions	History of cerebrovascular disease
Pregnancy	Peptic ulceration
Large left atrium with atrial fibrillation	Severe hypertension
	Oesophageal varices
	Heavy vaginal bleeding

The principal concern with thrombolysis is the risk of bleeding complications, as the drugs do not merely dissolve the clots at which they are aimed. Haemorrhagic stroke occurs in 0.5–1% of patients (NICE 2002a). However, the risk/benefit ratio remains in favour of administration in most cases and much has been made of targets that aim to speed thrombolytic administration (DoH 2003). The National Service Framework (DoH 2000a) outlines targets for the administration of thrombolysis: 75% of eligible patients were expected to receive treatment within 30 minutes of hospital arrival by April 2002, decreasing to 20 minutes by April 2003. A number of initiatives, including out-of-hospital thrombolysis (Quinn *et al.* 2002) and nurse-initiated thrombolysis (Wilmshurst *et al.* 2000), have been introduced in an attempt to reduce the time from presentation to initiation of treatment.

Continuous observation, including cardiac monitoring, is vital as cardiac arrest, particularly due to ventricular fibrillation (VF)/ventricular tachycardia (VT), can occur suddenly. However, if detected and treated quickly, the survival rate for cardiac arrest in these patients is high (Spearpoint *et al.* 2000) – up to 95% for patients in the first minute of VF (Bossaert 1997). Patients with ACS should be transferred to an appropriate clinical area without delay, usually the coronary care unit, accompanied by appropriate personnel and equipment.

RECOGNISING THE DETERIORATING PATIENT

Recognising a patient who is becoming or about to become seriously unwell, for any reason, has often relied on the nurse's intuition (Hams 2000) and unspecified 'concern' remains a valid reason for calling for help (Buist *et al.* 2002). However, in recent years there has been an emphasis on a systematic approach to patient assessment and the calling of rapid medical assistance based on objective criteria.

Similar to the assessment of a collapsed patient, immediate assessment of an acutely ill patient is based on the ABCDE system (Ahern & Philpott 2002, Anderson 1999, Smith 2003).

A   Airway
B   Breathing

C Circulation
D Disability
E Exposure

Patient assessment should only proceed to the next letter following full assessment and any necessary treatment from the previous one. For example, a blocked airway should be treated urgently; progression to assessment of breathing should occur only when the airway is open. Assessment includes the use of clinical assessment tools and monitoring with available equipment, though monitoring equipment should augment rather than replace assessment skills.

A = Airway
The airway can become obstructed for many reasons including:

- blood
- vomit
- a foreign body
- central nervous system depression
- bronchospasm
- laryngospasm (Resuscitation Council UK 2000).

In complete airway obstruction there are no breath sounds. If the patient is attempting to breathe there will be a seesaw (paradoxical) breathing pattern, with the abdomen moving in as the chest wall moves out during attempted inspiration. In the unconscious patient, obstruction of the pharynx by the tongue is the most common cause of complete airway obstruction. This is commonly, but inaccurately, known as 'swallowing the tongue' and occurs as muscle tone is lost. If the airway cannot be opened and cleared quickly by the use of the simple techniques described in Chapter 7, expert help must be summoned immediately.

Breathing is often noisy in partial airway obstruction. A conscious patient may be able to indicate that there is something wrong and there is often considerable distress. Treatment is directed at the cause and may involve simple airway opening manoeuvres with adjuncts and patient positioning, such as the recovery position. If there is no improvement or if advanced techniques, for example tracheal intubation, are required, senior help should be summoned without delay.

B = Breathing

If the airway is open, breathing can be assessed. There are many simple ways of assessing breathing.

• Counting the rate of respiration. Despite this being a very useful indicator of respiratory function (Smith 2003) that is easily and objectively measured, respiratory rates are often not counted (Kenward *et al.* 2001). The normal rate is between 12 and 20 breaths per minute, though this can vary between patients. Comparison with previously recorded observations is useful.

• Talking to a conscious patient. An extremely breathless patient may be unable to talk or manage only single words.

• Observing the respiratory pattern. Is chest movement symmetrical? Are accessory muscles in the neck and abdomen being used? How deep are the breaths?

• Looking for signs of cyanosis, such as bluish lips, but be aware that this is a delayed sign of impaired breathing (Smith 2003).

More detailed examinations, including feeling and listening to the chest and taking arterial blood for blood gas estimation, can be undertaken by a skilled practitioner.

Pulse oximetry

Pulse oximetry works by detecting absorption of red and infrared light as it passes through tissue, usually a fingertip (Moore 2004). Pulse oximetry is a useful non-invasive method which provides an indication of arterial oxygen saturation (SaO_2) and heart rate and can detect hypoxaemia. In health, the normal range for SaO_2 is 95–100%, although this may be lower for people with chronic respiratory problems. A sudden fall in SaO_2 in the presence of supplemental oxygen requires attention, as would a gradual decrease in levels. The probe must be cleaned prior to use and applied in an appropriate extremity such as finger or earlobe (also see Chapter 12). However, there are problems associated with the use of pulse oximeters in ill patients.

• There is often peripheral shutdown which makes the readings inaccurate.

• Cardiac rhythm abnormalities, such as atrial fibrillation, can alter readings.

- Oxygen saturation is not a reliable indicator of oxygen transport. Its values should be assessed in the light of other observations (Casey 2001).
- Pulse oximetry will not detect rising carbon dioxide levels and so a high SaO_2 can offer a false sense of security. A patient receiving supplemental oxygen can have a normal SaO_2 even when respiratory arrest is imminent.

Treatment
Treatment of breathlessness includes:

- supporting the patient by sitting in an upright position to reduce the work of breathing and enable the lungs to expand;
- administering oxygen;
- administering nebulisers as prescribed;
- treatment directed at the cause, e.g. diamorphine and frusemide for heart failure;
- non-invasive positive pressure ventilation (continuous positive airway pressure, CPAP) via a tightly fitting mask.

If these are not successful the patient may require invasive ventilation. This will normally require endotracheal intubation (see Chapter 7) and transfer to an intensive care unit.

Oxygen therapy
Oxygen is a drug and should be prescribed. However, it is recognised that often prescriptions are at best incomplete (Bateman & Leach 1998, Howell 2001). The principal aim of early treatment in acutely ill patients is the delivery of sufficient oxygen to the tissues (Puthucheary *et al.* 2002) and in the presence of impaired breathing, this will require supplemental oxygen. There is an understandable but overstated reluctance to give high dosages of oxygen. This is especially so where there is a history of chronic obstructive pulmonary disease (COPD). In type II respiratory failure, the concern is that patients who rely on a hypoxic respiratory drive will retain further carbon dioxide and develop respiratory acidosis or respiratory arrest if oxygen is given in too high a dose. However, type II respiratory failure occurs in only 10–15% of patients with COPD (Bateman & Leach 1998) and the small risk of hypercapnia must be

considered alongside the almost inevitable hypoxaemia that will result if sufficient oxygen is not given. Oxygen should never be withheld from an obviously hypoxic patient (Jevon & Ewens 2001).

All patients who are given oxygen therapy should be observed and monitored by pulse oximetry and arterial blood gases. Hypercapnia should be detected and addressed before it becomes dangerous. However, patients can and do die from hypoxia (Smith 2003).

Oxygen delivery

Oxygen can be delivered in a number of ways. Nasal cannulae deliver up to 40% oxygen but are more useful for long-term, low-rate administration and cannot deliver the concentrations required in the emergency situation.

Oxygen is most commonly given by facemasks and their function must be understood. However, lack of knowledge about oxygen and its delivery in both nurses and doctors has been demonstrated (Cooper 2002). A selection of facemasks is illustrated in Figures 2.4–2.7 which show:

- non-rebreathe mask. This mask uses a reservoir bag to enable high concentrations (approaching 100%) to be given (Smith 2003);
- humidified oxygen. The advantages of this system are that varying high concentrations can be delivered and that the oxygen will be humidified, preventing mucosal drying. However, it requires some equipment for assembly;
- Venturi masks. These masks regulate the concentration of oxygen by use of different coloured adaptors. The flow rate must be accurately set to deliver the set concentration;
- simple facemask. This can deliver up to 50–60% oxygen but the concentration can only be approximated.

C = Circulation

A failure to perfuse vital organs can lead to permanent damage and death. A rapid assessment of the circulation is therefore vital. Commonly performed assessments of circulation include pulse and blood pressure measurement.

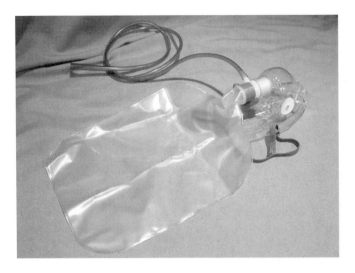

Fig. 2.4 A non-rebreathe mask.

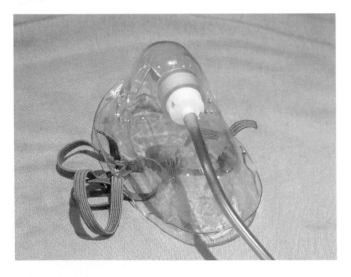

Fig. 2.5 A simple facemask.

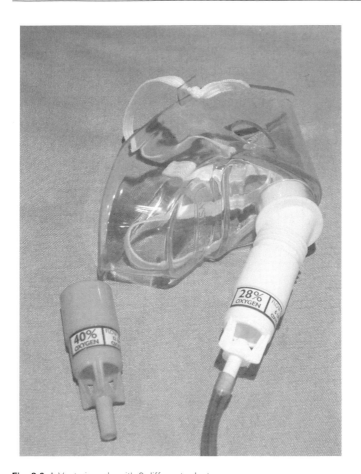

Fig. 2.6 A Venturi mask, with 2 different adaptors.

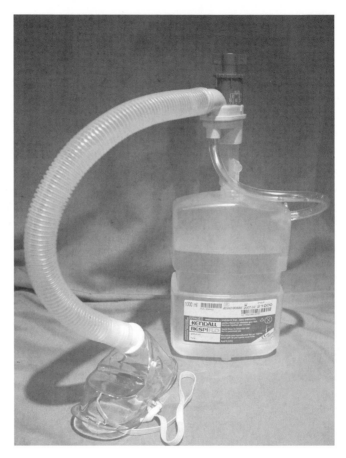

Fig. 2.7 A facemask using humidified oxygen.

Pulse

In the acutely ill patient, a rising pulse rate is often the first sign of impaired circulation, increased via the sympathetic nervous system as a result of falling blood pressure detected by baro-receptors in the neck and the aortic arch (Hinchliffe *et al.* 1996). The following should be noted.

- Rate. Normal can be considered as between 60 and 100 bpm, though as this varies between individuals, changes in the recorded trend rather than one-off values are important.
- Volume. A thin thready pulse with cool peripheries can indicate low cardiac output, e.g. hypovolaemia. A full, bounding pulse with warm peripheries can indicate sepsis.
- Regularity. An irregular pulse can indicate cardiac rhythm abnormalities.
- Pulse symmetry. Feel the pulse on both the left and right sides. A difference can suggest thoracic dissection.

Blood pressure

The measurement of blood pressure is commonly undertaken and yet there is evidence that nurses are unaware of how it is best performed (Armstrong 2002). It remains an important measure of critical illness, though a reduction in blood pressure from baseline values is often a delayed sign of shock, as heart rate and force of contraction and peripheral vasoconstriction act to normalise blood pressure.

It is important that the correct equipment is used to measure blood pressure. Automated machines have become common though not all have been independently validated (Feather 2001). They have some advantages but also limitations; cuff size is vitally important for determining accurate blood pressure and a recent study found that more than 30% of measurements by oscillometric blood pressure machine in critically ill patients were outside a clinically accepted range of accuracy (Bur *et al*. 2003). Automated machines may also fail to detect variations in pulse, such as atrial fibrillation.

Other ways of assessing circulation include:

- looking at and feeling the patient, who may be pale and sweaty, have cool limbs, be acting abnormally and have poor urine output;
- the capillary refill time (CRT) may be prolonged, showing sluggish peripheral circulation. Press the skin on the fingertip for five seconds and release. The skin should be blanched on release of the pressure but the colour should return within two seconds (Ahern & Philpott 2002);
- looking for obvious signs of haemorrhage.

Hypotension is a medical emergency. There are a number of causes of hypotension (Smith 2003), but most will require rapid administration of intravenous fluids.

D = Disability

Many acutely ill patients have changes in their conscious level. A major concern in a patient whose conscious level is deteriorating is protection of the airway and so the patient should not be left alone if at all possible. There are many reasons why a patient's conscious level may deteriorate. It may simply be a result of decreased cerebral perfusion. A full neurological examination may be helpful. However, for the purposes of rapid assessment of responsiveness in the acutely ill patients, the AVPU scale is commonly used.

A   Alert
V   Responds to voice
P   Responds to pain
U   Unresponsive

E = Exposure

Exposure refers to the necessity for a full visual physical inspection and examination of the patient. For example, there may not be an obvious sign of bleeding or of injury, therefore it is important to examine the patient from head to toe, front and back.

TRIGGERING ASSISTANCE

Studies similar to those demonstrating that most cardiac arrests are avoidable have shown that early recognition of deterioration and admission to an intensive care unit dramatically improves survival rates of acutely ill patients (McQuillan *et al.* 1998). Unfortunately deterioration often goes unnoticed or is treated inappropriately (McQuillan *et al.* 1998). This recognition has led to a number of initiatives (DoH 2000b):

- education, especially for ward-based staff (Smith *et al.* 2002);
- support for general wards from critical care units (Coombs & Dillon 2002);
- systems for calling specialist clinicians before cardiac arrest.

A delay by nursing staff in informing medical staff of deterioration in a patient's condition is a common feature of avoidable cardiac arrests (Hodgetts *et al.* 2002a), and has been so for a number of years (Franklin & Mathew 1994). A number of systems for reporting deterioration are in operation.

Medical emergency team (METS)

METS were developed in the mid-1990s (Hourihan *et al.* 1995) and have been implemented in some trusts in the UK (Hodgetts *et al.* 2002b). In this scheme a team of specialists is called in response to certain clinical criteria. The team then manages the patient on the ward and arranges transfer if appropriate. A variation is where the cardiac arrest team is called prior to cardiac arrest occurring. An example of calling criteria is patient unrousable AND one or more of the following:

- respiration rate less than 7 or more than 40 bpm
- heart rate less than 35 or more than 180 bpm
- systolic blood pressure less than 65 mmHg
- oxygen saturation less than 85% (Gloucestershire Hospitals NHS Trust 2003).

Early warning systems (EWS)

This approach differs in that the patient's own team is called in response to clinical criteria interpreted in a scoring system. The team must attend within a certain time according to an algorithm. The precise values for the scoring system vary between hospitals. Some include urine output as a variable (Carberry 2002, Sterling & Groba 2002). Table 2.2 shows the scoring criteria at Gloucestershire Hospitals NHS Trust. Figure 2.8 shows the algorithm.

Critical care outreach

Critical care outreach teams, often headed by a consultant nurse, have become common in the UK (McArthur-Rose 2001). Their precise remits vary between hospitals. Most are available for education and advice and nurses should be aware of the personnel and the remit of the team in individual hospitals.

Table 2.2 Early warning system calling criteria.

Score	3	2	1	0	1	2	3
Temp (°C)		<35	35–35.9	36–37.9	38–38.9	>39	
Systolic BP	<70	71–80	81–100	101–199		>200	
Heart rate		<40	41–50	51–100	101–110	111–139	>140
Respiratory rate		<8		9–14	15–20	21–29	>30
CNS			New agitation or confusion	Alert	Voice		Pain Unresponsive

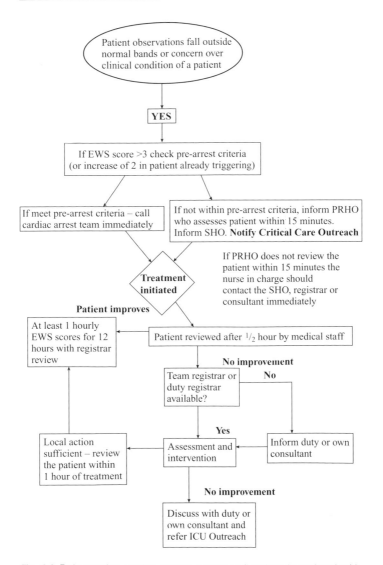

Fig. 2.8 Early warning scoring system treatment flowchart (reproduced with permission from Gloucestershire Hospitals NHS Trust).

COMMUNICATION

Communication between healthcare professionals is especially important when caring for an acutely ill patient. Particularly important are:

- the need for accurate clinical information. A completed assessment should be available when telephoning for help;
- assertiveness in calling for help from more senior staff when needed;
- the requirement for clear documentation and a management plan. The instruction 'Give fluids and call Dr if urine output falls' is useless. Clear instructions should be provided. 'If urine output is less than 30 ml per hour for 2 consecutive hours, give 500 ml of normal saline and inform medical registrar on call.'
- it is vital to keep the patient and relatives informed in clear, jargon-free language (Smith 2003).

REVIEW OF LEARNING

- ❏ Most cardiac arrests are avoidable if recognised and treated early.
- ❏ Most cardiac arrests are associated with ACS or related symptoms.
- ❏ Treatment for ACS depends on the clinical history, presentation of symptoms, risk factors, ECG changes and cardiac enzyme increase.
- ❏ Treatment of NSTEMI and STEMI needs to be rapid.
- ❏ Recognising the acutely ill patient requires skill and knowledge of how to perform a systematic clinical assessment and identify priorities.
- ❏ Assessment of patients whose condition is deteriorating must include Airway, Breathing, Circulation, Disability and Exposure.
- ❏ Early warning systems, if appropriately used, can provide evidence of a deterioration in a patient's condition.
- ❏ Healthcare professionals should be aware of local procedures for summoning expert assistance based on EWS scores.

CONCLUSION

Recognising and responding to the early signs and symptoms in the patient who is critically ill and at risk of a cardiac arrest demands skilled systematic assessment of vital functions in order to intervene appropriately. Nurses at the bedside are most likely to identify this group of vulnerable patients and therefore their assessment and actions will be of vital significance in preventing many avoidable deaths.

REFERENCES

Ahern, J. & Philpott, P. (2002) Assessing acutely ill patients on general wards. *Nursing Standard* **16** (47), 47–56.

Albarran, J. (2002) The language of chest pain. *Nursing Times* **98** (4), 38–9.

Albarran, J.W. & Kapeluch, H. (2000) Role of the nurse in thrombolytic therapy – expanding the clinical horizons. In: Cruickshank, J.P., Bradbury, M. & Ashurst, S. (eds) *Aspects of Cardiovascular Nursing*. BJN monograph. Mark Allen Publishing, Dinton.

Anderson, I.D. (ed.) (1999) *Care of the Critically Ill Surgical Patient*. Arnold, London.

Armstrong, R. (2002) Nurses' knowledge of error in blood pressure recording technique. *International Journal of Nursing Practice* **8** (3), 118–26.

Baron, J.H., Joy, A. & Millar-Craig, M. (2004) How do we define myocardial infarction? A survey of the views of consultant physicians and cardiologists. *British Journal of Cardiology* **11**, 34–8.

Bateman, N.T. & Leach, R.M. (1998) ABC of oxygen: acute oxygen therapy. *British Medical Journal* **317** (7161), 798–801.

Bossaert, L.L. (1997) Fibrillation and defibrillation of the heart. *British Journal of Anaesthesia* **79**, 203–13.

British Cardiac Society and Medical Practice Committee, Royal College of Physicians Clinical Effectiveness and Evaluation Unit (2001) Guideline for the management of patients with acute coronary syndrome without persistent ECG ST segment elevation. *Heart* **85** (2), 133–42.

British National Formulary (2003) Available online at: www.bnf.org

Buist, M.D., Moore, G.E., Bernard, S.A., Waxman, B.P., Anderson, J.N. & Nguyen, T.V. (2002) Effects of a medical emergency team on reduction of incidence of and mortality from unexpected cardiac arrests in hospital: preliminary study. *British Medical Journal* **324** (7334), 387–90.

Bur, A., Herkner, H., Vlcek, M. *et al.* (2003) Factors influencing the accuracy of oscillometric blood pressure measurement in critically ill patients. *Critical Care Medicine* **31** (3), 793–9.

Carberry, M. (2002) Implementing the modified early warning system: our experiences. *Nursing in Critical Care* **7** (5), 220–6.

Casey, G. (2001) Oxygen transport and the use of pulse oximetry. *Nursing Standard* **15** (47), 46–55.

Coombs, M. & Dillon, A. (2002) Crossing boundaries, re-defining care: the role of the critical care outreach team. *Journal of Clinical Nursing* **11**, 387–93.

Cooper, N. (2002) Oxygen therapy – myths and misconceptions. *Care of the Critically Ill* **18** (3), 74–7.

Davies, M.J. (2000) The pathophysiology of acute coronary syndromes. *Heart* **83** (3), 361–6.

Department of Health (2000a) *National Service Framework for Coronary Heart Disease.* Department of Health, London.

Department of Health (2000b) *Comprehensive Critical Care – A Review of Adult Critical Care Services.* Department of Health, London.

Department of Health (2003) *Review of Early Thrombolysis – Faster and Better Treatment for Heart Attack Patients.* Department of Health, London.

Domanovits, H., Schillinger, M., Paulis, M. *et al.* (2002) Acute chest pain – a stepwise approach. The challenge of the correct clinical diagnosis. *Resuscitation* **55**, 9–16.

Edwards, S.L. (2002) Myocardial infarction: the nursing responsibilities in the first hour. *British Journal of Nursing* **11** (7), 454–68.

Feather, C. (2001) Equipment for blood pressure measurement. *Professional Nurse* **16** (11), 1458–62.

Franklin, C. & Mathew, J. (1994) Developing strategies to prevent inhospital cardiac arrest: analysing responses of physicians and nurses in the hours before the event. *Critical Care Medicine* **22** (2), 244–7.

Galvani, M., Ottani, F., Ferrini, D. *et al.* (1997) Prognostic influence of elevated values of cardiac troponin I in patients with unstable angina. *Circulation* **95** (8), 2053–9.

Gerschlick, A.H. (2001) The acute management of myocardial infarction. In: Gerschlick, A.H. & Davies, S.W. (eds) *Ischaemic Heart Disease: Therapeutic Issues.* British Medical Bulletin 59. Oxford University Press, Oxford.

Gloucestershire Hospitals NHS Trust (2003) *Revised Cardiac Arrest Calling Criteria.* Gloucestershire Hospitals NHS Trust, Gloucester.

Hams, S.P. (2000) A gut feeling? Intuition and critical care nursing. *Intensive and Critical Care Nursing* **16**, 310–18.

Hand, H. (2001) Myocardial infarction: part 1. *Nursing Standard* **15** (36), 45–55.

Harrison, H. (1999) Troponin I. *American Journal of Nursing* **99** (5), 24TT–24VV.

Hinchliffe, S.M., Montague, S.E. & Watson, R. (1996) *Physiology for Nursing Practice*, 2nd edn. Baillière Tindall, London.

Hodgetts, T.J., Kenward, G., Vlackonikolis, I. *et al.* (2002a) Incidence, location and reasons for avoidable in-hospital cardiac arrest in a district general hospital. *Resuscitation* **54**, 115–23.

Hodgetts, T.J., Kenward, G., Vlackonikolis, I.G., Payne, S. & Castle, N. (2002b) The identification of risk factors for cardiac arrest and formulation of activation criteria to alert a medical emergency team. *Resuscitation* **54**, 125–31.

Hourihan, F., Bishop, G., Hillman, K.M., Daffurn, K. & Lee, A. (1995) The medical emergency team: a new strategy to identify and intervene in high risk patients. *Clinical Intensive Care* **6**, 269–72.

Howell, M. (2001) An audit of oxygen prescribing in acute general medical wards. *Professional Nurse* **17** (4), 221–4.

Hughes, K. (2003) Pharmacological treatment of acute coronary syndromes. *Professional Nurse* **18** (5), 296–9.

Jevon, P. (2003) *ECGs for Nurses*. Blackwell Publishing, Oxford.

Jevon, P. & Ewens, B. (2001) Assessment of a breathless patient. *Nursing Standard* **15** (16), 48–55.

Jones, I. (2003) Acute coronary syndromes: identification and patient care. *Professional Nurse* **18** (5), 289–92.

Jowett, N.I. & Thompson, D.R. (2003) *Comprehensive Coronary Care*, 3rd edn. Baillière Tindall, Edinburgh.

Kenward, G., Hodgetts, T. & Castle, N. (2001) Time to put the R back in TPR. *Nursing Times* **97** (40), 32–3.

McArthur-Rose, F. (2001) Critical care outreach services and early warning scoring systems: a review of the literature. *Journal of Advanced Nursing* **36** (5), 696–704.

McQuillan, P., Pilkington, S., Allan, A. *et al.* (1998) Confidential inquiry into quality of care before admission to intensive care. *British Medical Journal* **316**, 1853–8.

Moore, T. (2004) *Pulse oximetry*. In: Moore, T. & Woodrow, P. (Eds) *High Dependency Nursing Care*. Routledge, London.

National Institute for Clinical Excellence (2002a) *Guidance on the Use of GlycoproteinIIa/IIIb Inhibitors in the Treatment of Acute Coronary Syndromes*. National Institute for Clinical Excellence, London.

National Institute for Clinical Excellence (2002b) *Guidance on the Use of Drugs for Early Thrombolysis in the Treatment of Acute Myocardial Infarction*. National Institute for Clinical Excellence, London.

Puthucheary, Z., Whitehead, M.A. & Grounds, M. (2002) Early management of the critically ill patient. *Clinical Medicine* **2** (2), 98–100.

Quinn, T., Butters, A. & Todd, I. (2002) Implementing paramedic thrombolysis: an overview. *Accident and Emergency Nursing* **10** (4), 189–96.

Resuscitation Council UK (2000) *Advanced Life Support Course Provider Manual*, 4th edn. Resuscitation Council UK, London.

Smith, A.F. & Wood, J. (1998) Can some in-hospital cardio-respiratory arrests be prevented? A prospective survey. *Resuscitation* **37**, 133–7.

Smith, G.B. (2003) *ALERT. A Multiprofessional Course in Care of the Acutely Ill*, 2nd edn. University of Portsmouth, Portsmouth.

Smith, G.B., Osgood, V.M., Crane, S. and the ALERT Course Development Group (2002) ALERT™ – a multiprofessional training course in the care of the acutely ill adult patient. *Resuscitation* **52**, 281–6.

Spearpoint, K.G., McClean, C.P. & Zideman, D.A. (2000) Early defibrillation and the chain of survival in 'in hospital' cardiac arrest: minutes count. *Resuscitation* **44** (3), 165–9.

Sterling, C. & Groba, C.B. (2002) An audit of a patient-at-risk trigger scoring system for identifying seriously ill ward patients. *Nursing in Critical Care* **7** (5), 215–19.

Stevens, M. (2002) Glycoprotein IIa/IIIb inhibitors. *Intensive and Critical Care Nursing* **18**, 64–6.

Wilmshurst, P., Purcase, A., Webb, A., Jowett, C. & Quinn, T. (2000) Improving door to needle times with nurse initiated thrombolysis. *Heart* **84** (3), 262–6.

Zipes, D.P. & Wellens, H.J.J. (1998) Sudden cardiac death. *Circulation* **98** (21), 2334–51.

Resuscitation Equipment

3

INTRODUCTION

The best possible chance of patient survival following a cardiac arrest in a clinical environment can only be given if the arrest is promptly recognised and responded to by staff who have received appropriate training and have essential emergency equipment available. Most general hospitals will organise their resuscitation equipment onto a trolley that is known as the 'cardiac arrest' or 'crash' trolley. Other hospitals or departments may assemble their equipment in the form of a 'grab bag' or a wall-mounted board or box. What must be remembered is the standard which states that, where indicated, all patients should be defibrillated within three minutes from the time of collapse in all areas of the hospital (Resuscitation Council UK 2000).

AIMS

This chapter considers equipment that is commonly used in a respiratory or cardiac arrest situation and outlines considerations regarding the maintenance of equipment.

LEARNING OUTCOMES

By the end of this chapter the reader should be able to:

❏ appreciate the way in which *cardiac arrest equipment may be organised*;
❏ list *essential resuscitation equipment* for dealing with a patient's airway, breathing and circulation;
❏ appreciate *other miscellaneous equipment* that may be required during a resuscitation attempt;
❏ outline their *individual responsibilities* with regard to resuscitation equipment.

THE CARDIAC ARREST TROLLEY

Cardiac arrest trolleys (or other system) should ideally be located in every clinical ward and department. The equipment placed upon them should be standardised throughout the hospital so that any attending cardiac arrest or emergency team member will be presented with the same system regardless of the ward or department they are responding to.

The hospital resuscitation officer (RO) will generally have responsibility for overseeing resuscitation equipment and its standardisation within their trust. Advice should always be sought from the RO before adding or removing a particular type of equipment from the system. The scenario of every ward or department putting together their own trolley or making their own mark on it should be avoided, as the attending team will require a standardised approach. There may be one or two exceptions to this rule, for example in maternity units where specific extra equipment may be required immediately as part of the resuscitation.

A laminated list of the contents of the trolley should be available and some kind of system established to ensure that the trolley content has been checked on a daily or weekly basis (and immediately after use). The defibrillator may be kept upon the top of this trolley. It should be noted that it is the responsibility of every healthcare professional to be familiar with the layout and contents of their organisation's trolley or system. One of the best ways to ensure familiarity is to regularly get involved in checking the trolley. Locum or agency staff should always be orientated to the location of the emergency equipment.

In addition to the standard equipment for managing airway, breathing and circulation, certain other items need to be portable and immediately available, for example oxygen and a suction machine.

Access will also be required for equipment that is not necessarily needed immediately during the resuscitation but will certainly be required post arrest, such as a blood pressure measuring device, a pulse oximeter and a 12-lead electrocardiograph (ECG) machine.

Resuscitation equipment

The Resuscitation Council UK (2001a) provides a list of recommended equipment for the management of adult cardiopulmonary arrest, as follows.

Airway and breathing equipment (see Figures 3.1 and 3.2)
- Pocket masks with oxygen port
- Self-inflating bag-valve with oxygen reservoir and tubing
- Clear facemasks sizes 4, 5 and 6
- Oropharyngeal airways sizes 2, 3 and 4
- Yankaeur suckers
- Endotracheal suction catheters × 10
- Laryngeal mask airway (size 4) or Combitube (small)
- Magill forceps
- Endotracheal tubes – oral, cuffed, sizes 6, 7 and 8
- Nasopharyngeal airways, sizes 6, 7 and 8
- Catheter mount
- Gum elastic bougie
- Lubricating jelly
- Laryngoscopes (ideally two, with normal and long blades)
- Spare laryngoscope bulbs and batteries
- 1″ (2.5 cm) ribbon gauze/tape
- Scissors
- Syringe – 20 ml
- Clear oxygen mask with reservoir bag, such as Hudson mask
- Oxygen supply
- Cylinder key

It is also suggested that the following are included:

- nasogastric tube;
- suction machine or manual device.

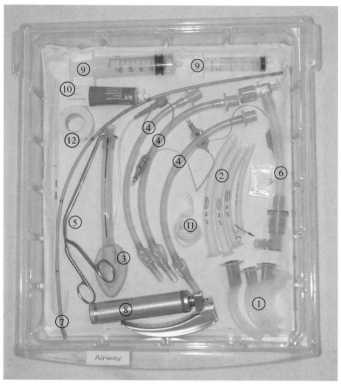

Index of equipment

1. Guedel airways
2. Nasopharyngeal airways
3. LMA
4. Endotracheal tubes (oral and cuffed)
5. McGill forceps
6. Catheter mount with swivel connector
7. Gum elastic bougie
8. Laryngoscope with curved blade (spare laryngoscope with blades should also be available)
9. Syringes (10 ml and 50 ml)
10. Lubricant
11. 1″ (2.5 cm) ribbon gauze or tape
12. Micropore

Fig. 3.1 Airway drawer of a cardiac arrest trolley (adult).

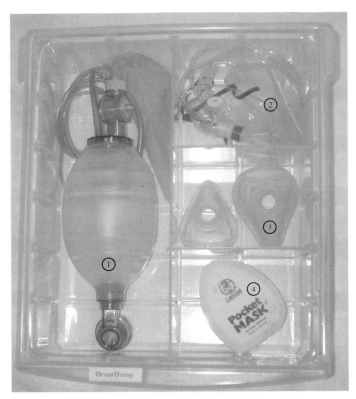

Index of equipment

1. Self-inflating resuscitation bag with oxygen reservoir and oxygen tubing
2. Clear oxygen facemask with reservoir bag
3. Clear facemask to be attached to (1)
4. Pocket mask used to deliver assisted breaths in the unconscious patient

Fig. 3.2 Breathing drawer of a cardiac arrest trolley (adult).

Circulation equipment
- Intravenous cannulae 18 gauge × 3, 14 gauge × 3
- Hypodermic needles 21 gauge × 10
- Syringes 2 ml × 6, 5 ml × 6, 10 ml × 6, 20 ml × 6

- Cannulae fixing dressings and tapes × 4
- Seldinger wire central line kits × 2
- 12-gauge central venous cannulae × 2
- Intravenous giving sets × 3
- 0.9% sodium chloride – 1000 ml × 2

It is also suggested that the following are included:

- razors;
- sharps box;
- defibrillator.

Drugs
Immediately available pre-filled syringes:

- adrenaline/epinephrine 1 mg (1 : 10 000) × 4
- atropine 3 mg × 1
- amiodarone 300 mg × 1.

Other readily available drugs:

- adrenaline/epinephrine 1 mg (1 : 10 000) × 4
- sodium bicarbonate 8.4% – 50 ml × 1
- calcium chloride 13.24% – 10 ml × 2
- lidocaine/lignocaine 100 mg × 2
- atropine 1 mg × 2
- normal saline 10 ml ampoules × 10
- naloxone 400 µg × 2
- adrenaline/epinephrine 1 : 1000 × 2
- amiodarone 150 mg × 4
- magnesium sulphate 50% solution 2 g (4 ml) × 1
- potassium chloride 40 mmol × 1
- adenosine 6 mg × 10
- midazolam 10 mg × 1
- hydrocortisone 200 mg × 1
- glucose 10% 500 ml × 1.

Additional items
- ECG electrodes
- Defibrillation gel pads
- Clock
- Gloves/goggles/aprons

It is good practice to have audit/cardiac arrest report forms in order to record, audit and learn from the experience.

Additionally, a sliding sheet or similar device should also be available for safer handling.

Equipment for the primary care environment

Due to the specific nature of the primary care environment, a separate document outlines the minimal equipment that should be available in such a setting (Resuscitation Council UK 2001b). This is basically a scaled-down version of the standard equipment noted above and takes into consideration the possibility of very few personnel being available to deal with the cardiac arrest. In many situations there may simply be one person to deal with the arrest.

In the hospital situation resuscitation equipment must be readily accessible and organised according to agreed protocols, often in a trolley system, with a defibrillator on the top.

Equipment for managing the airway

Contents of the airway drawer will vary; indeed, some systems may not identify this section of their trolley or bag as 'airway'. Often the airway and breathing are considered to be the same thing and equipment such as a pocket mask may be found in the airway drawer as opposed to the breathing drawer. Figure 3.1 is an example of how the 'airway drawer' may be set out. With this particular type of trolley system, each drawer can actually be removed from the trolley, so the airway drawer, for example, may be passed up to the head of the patient to allow the healthcare professional managing the airway easier access to the equipment they are likely to require. The drawers also have a plastic lid type cover to them (not shown), which works well in preventing the accumulation of dust on the equipment.

Oropharyngeal airways

- This is often referred to as a *Guedel airway*™ (see Figure 3.1, item 1).
- It is a plastic, curved tube, with a reinforced section and flange at the oral end. The reinforced section is a bite block

and is designed to sit between the teeth. The remainder of the tube fits between the tongue and posterior pharyngeal wall.

- The oral airway can only be used in patients who are unconscious or sedated with no gag reflex. It will cause gagging or straining in a patient whose reflex responses are intact. Such a patient may be a suitable candidate for a nasopharyngeal airway.
- The oropharyngeal airway comes in a range of sizes to fit newborns up to large adults.
- For guidelines on sizing and insertion, see Chapter 7.

Nasopharyngeal airways

- Designed to help maintain a patent airway. They are indicated in the patient who is not deeply unconscious and therefore unable to tolerate an oropharyngeal airway, yet needs a simple adjunct to help maintain airway patency.
- Nasopharyngeal airways are soft, flexible plastic tubes with an angular end and a trumpet-shaped end.
- They may be particularly useful in patients with maxillofacial injuries or in situations where it is impossible to open the patient's mouth (clenched or wired jaws, trismus).
- This device is best avoided in a patient with a base-of-skull fracture for fear of intracranial insertion.
- For guidelines on sizing and insertion, see Chapter 7.

Laryngeal mask airway (LMA)

The LMA is an adjunctive airway composed of a wide-bore tube with an elliptical inflatable cuff that, when inflated, provides a seal around the laryngeal opening (see Figure 3.1, item 3). The LMA is an extremely reliable device that can be used during a resuscitation attempt by nurses and other paramedical staff who may not be skilled in endotracheal intubation (Anonymous 1994). It is important, as with any piece of equipment, that the operator has undergone the necessary training and assessment procedures as outlined by their place of work.

For guidelines on sizing and insertion, see Chapter 7.

Endotracheal tube (ETT)

- Designed to offer full protection in securing the patient's airway. Considered to be the 'gold standard' in maintaining an airway.
- The cuffed tube is inserted directly into the trachea under clear and direct vision using a laryngoscope.
- Prior to inflation of the cuff, the operator checks for correct tube placement by auscultation of the lungs with a stethoscope.
- The ETT may be attached directly to a ventilation device such as a bag-valve system with or without oxygen attached.
- A fine-bore suction catheter may be inserted through the ETT to remove secretions, etc. from the lower airways.
- The ETT is an alternative route for drug delivery in the event of intravenous access (IV) access not being achieved.

McGill forceps

- Forceps with long angled levers designed to assist in removing objects or foreign bodies from the patient's airway, for example a dislodged denture plate.
- They may also be used in assisting intubation.

Catheter mount with swivel connector

- Designed to fit between the end connection port of an ETT, LMA or Combitube (see Chapter 7) and the bag-valve ventilation system.
- The catheter mount gives an extra bit of leeway between the bag and any tube, generally resulting in less possibility of dislodging a tube.
- An added bonus is that a port on top of the catheter mount will allow the passage of a soft suction catheter down through the tube to remove any secretions. This can be performed without having to disconnect the bag from the tube on each occasion, hence reducing the risk of dislodging the tube.

Introducers

- Two types of introducers are shown in Figure 3.1, item 7. There is a rigid introducer (or stylet) and a gum elastic flexible introducer, known as a bougie.

- During intubation the rigid introducer may be used inside an ETT to alter the natural curvature of the tube dependent on the patient's airway anatomy.
- The bougie can also aid in difficult intubation but this tends to be inserted into the airway first and the ETT would then be slipped over the bougie and into the correct place using the bougie as a guide.

Laryngoscope

- The laryngoscope (see Figure 3.1, item 8) is a device generally used for intubation and to give direct clear vision of a patient's oropharynx. It may have other uses, such as providing a light source during the removal of foreign material.
- During daily or weekly checking of the trolley, the blade of the laryngoscope should be pulled up to a 90° angle and locked in place to assess the brightness of the light source and battery function.
- Different sized blades are recommended although for most adult patients a size 3 Macintosh blade will suffice.
- It is a good idea to have a second laryngoscope on the trolley in the event of failure of the first.
- Spare batteries and bulbs (if it is not of a fibreoptic type) should always be available on the trolley.

Miscellaneous

There are other things which will be necessary in airway management, such as:

- lubricating jelly – to assist in nasopharyngeal, LMA or ETT insertion;
- tape or ribbon gauze – to tie in or secure an airway device such as an LMA or ETT;
- syringe – airway devices such as the ETT and LMA will require inflation with air. An LMA, dependent on size, may require up to 40 ml of air to be inserted.

More information on the use of airway equipment may be found in Chapter 7.

Equipment for managing breathing

Figure 3.2 is an example of how the 'breathing drawer' of a cardiac arrest trolley may be laid out. In some departments, the bag-valve-mask system may be found readily attached to the oxygen and in a more accessible location, where it can be seen hooked on the drip stand. However, if it is located in the drawer as indicated below, it is less likely to accumulate dust.

Bag-valve system

This system is often referred to as the 'Ambu-Bag'™. It consists of a self-inflating bag and a one-way non-rebreathing valve. When the bag is squeezed the air is delivered to the patient's lungs via the one-way valve. On releasing the squeeze, the bag self-inflates with room air that enters via an inlet at the opposite end of the bag. When oxygen becomes available, a reservoir bag should be attached to this inlet and the oxygen flow set at 10–15l/min. The patient's exhaled air is released back into the atmosphere by the one-way valve and does not contaminate the contents of the bag. The bag-valve device may be used with a facemask, a laryngeal mask airway, an endotracheal tube or a Combitube (Resuscitation Council UK 2000).

Pocket mask

- The pocket mask is a facemask that allows mouth-to-mask ventilation of the patient (see Figure 3.2, item 4).
- It is available with or without an inlet that allows additional oxygen to be attached. Preferably one with an oxygen inlet should be used in the hospital setting.
- The pocket mask is available in one size for adults and will allow a good seal in most casualties.
- For guidelines on sizing and insertion, see Chapter 7.

Non-rebreathe oxygen masks

- For the patient who is spontaneously breathing, an oxygen mask should be available (see Figure 3.2, item 2).
- The non-rebreathe oxygen mask has a reservoir bag attached, allowing an oxygen concentration of about 85% when delivered at a flow rate of 10–15l/min.

More information on the use of ventilation equipment may be found in Chapter 7.

Equipment for managing the circulation

Intravenous connectors and three-way taps
- A selection of connectors is necessary for any IV infusions that may be commenced.
- Three-way taps are often connected between a giving set and the patient's IV access so that a syringe can be attached, allowing boluses of saline to be drawn from the bag and pushed into the IV line following administration of any drug bolus.

Giving sets and air inlets
- A giving set may be required for the administration of IV fluid.
- Dependent on the IV fluid container type, an air inlet (wide-bore needles with special filter) may need to be inserted into the container to increase the rate of fluid administration.

Selection of hypodermic needles
- Several needles may be required for the drawing up of cardiac arrest drugs that are sometimes not available in pre-filled syringes. They may also be required for drawing up saline boluses if the method suggested above is not used.
- Blood gas syringes may be located in this drawer also.

Razors, 12-lead ECG electrodes and normal ECG monitoring electrodes
- It is always useful to have several razors available in case the patient's chest is very hairy, resulting in ECG electrodes that fail to adhere properly to the chest wall.
- The ECG electrodes should be replaced on the trolley regularly as once removed from their packet, the gel within the electrode may dry out and result in an electrode not sticking to the chest wall in an emergency.

Intravenous cannulae
Early access to the circulation is important in cardiac arrest so that drugs can be administered quickly. A selection of large-bore cannulae should be available.

IV cannulae dressing
In an emergency, normal surgical tape can be used to secure a cannula in place but having a proper IV cannulae dressing will offer extra security against any IV access accidentally being dislodged.

Water/normal saline for injection
Saline boluses may be given directly from a bag of saline connected to the IV line by a giving set. However, if this option is not employed then normal 20 ml ampoules are required. Water for injection may be necessary for drawing up some types of drugs.

Scissors
A pair of heavy-duty scissors may be required to cut through some types of clothing and gain access to the chest so that defibrillation can be performed quickly.

Tourniquet
Gaining IV access is often difficult in a cardiac arrest situation. In an emergency, one member of the team may use their hands to form a tourniquet around the patient's limb whilst another team member is inserting the cannula. However, this does not offer an even tourniquet pressure and therefore use of a proper tourniquet is more desirable.

Gauze and surgical tape
• Gauze pads may be required to cover any bleeding sites, for example following blood gas analysis or removal of a cannula.
• Surgical tape may be used to secure gauze in place or to secure an airway device, for example an ETT.

Further information on IV access and drug delivery can be found in Chapter 10 and more information on ECG monitoring and defibrillation may be found in Chapters 8 and 9.

Drugs and fluids

Drugs and fluids may be considered part of the equipment needed for circulation and many hospitals will have specific 'cardiac arrest drug boxes'. These are often separated down further into 'first-line' and 'second-line' drugs. The list recommended by the Resuscitation Council UK (2001a) is very comprehensive, particularly the section on 'other readily available drugs'. This could be interpreted as 'second-line' drugs and whilst desirable, it is not absolutely necessary to keep all of these on the trolley, particularly if space is limited. In this case, the second-line drugs should be kept together in an appropriate location that is easily and rapidly accessible.

Intravenous fluids

- There has been lengthy debate regarding the best type of fluid to be given in emergency situations. Most cardiac arrest trolleys will stock both a crystalloid (such as 0.9% normal saline) and a colloid (such as gelofusin).
- A bag of 5% dextrose is often kept on the trolley as, if prefilled syringes are not available, this is the medium generally used if diluting the drug amiodarone.

Pre-filled drug syringes

There are two different pre-filled drug systems in general use in the UK – the Min-I-Jet™ system and the Aurum™ system. Please see Chapter 10 for advice on the assembly and use of these systems.

Miscellaneous equipment

A miscellaneous drawer is useful for storing essential equipment that may be too bulky or cumbersome or just take up a lot of space in one of the other drawers; for example, spare oxygen masks, laryngoscope bulbs and spares.

Suction catheters

- Any suction device is likely to have a rigid suction catheter already attached to it but several spare catheters should be on the trolley.
- A selection of fine-bore flexible catheters should also be available.

• These catheters may be more appropriately placed in the airway drawer, depending on available space.

Spare canister for the suction apparatus
As it is possible that arrests may occur sequentially with no time for restocking of the trolley, it is most useful to have at least one spare of everything.

Gloves/goggles/aprons
The use of personal protective equipment during a cardiac arrest situation is strongly recommended, particularly the use of gloves as contact with body fluids is very likely.

Defibrillation gel pads
Often the defibrillation gel pads are stored on top of the defibrillator, so that they are immediately obvious to the operator. However, the defibrillator, when attached to the mains in charging mode, will generate a very small amount of warmth and this may dry out the gel pads. Storing them elsewhere is therefore recommended.

INDIVIDUAL RESPONSIBILITIES
Every healthcare practitioner has a responsibility to be familiar with cardiac arrest equipment. Practical training in the use of resuscitation equipment is likely to be available through the hospital RO. Whilst familiarity is required by all healthcare professionals, training in the actual use of a piece of equipment may not be appropriate; for example, using a laryngoscope and ETT to intubate a patient is a very specialist skill.

Following a resuscitation attempt, it is important that the cardiac arrest trolley or system is replenished almost immediately in case a further cardiac arrest occurs in a short time frame.

Equipment such as the LMA may be disposable or autoclavable. However, many items of resuscitation equipment are now completely disposable after single use.

It is always worth considering what would happen in the event of equipment failure and where alternative equipment may be found. Following a resuscitation event, any faulty equipment should be reported and replaced.

REVIEW OF LEARNING

❏ Resuscitation equipment should be available to all departments and wards.

❏ This should include airway, breathing and circulation equipment and drugs.

❏ The equipment should be organised systematically for easy access.

❏ All resuscitation equipment should be checked daily and following arrests.

❏ Every healthcare practitioner should be familiar with the cardiac arrest equipment.

Case study

Review and consider the answers to the following questions.

- **Are you familiar with and able to identify the contents of your cardiac arrest trolley or system?**

- **Do you know where to seek further training in your organisation?**

- **Do you know how to replenish the trolley after it has been used?**

- **Do you know which equipment is disposable and which needs to be cleaned and disinfected, either locally or centrally?**

- **Do you know what to do in the event of equipment failure?**

There are no answers provided, as you need to know the system that is particular to your individual organisation. If you are uncertain on any aspect then you have a professional responsibility to seek clarity.

CONCLUSION

It is imperative that every healthcare practitioner is familiar with any equipment that they may have to use in an emergency.

A cardiac arrest is almost always a stressful situation and lack of knowledge or familiarity with equipment and procedures will only increase the pressures of the event and is likely to delay appropriate interventions for the patient.

REFERENCES
Anonymous (1994) The use of the laryngeal mask airway by nurses during cardiopulmonary resuscitation – results of a multicentre trial. *Anaesthesia* **49** (1), 3–7.

Resuscitation Council UK (2000) *Advanced Life Support Course Provider Manual*, 4th edn. Resuscitation Council UK, London.

Resuscitation Council UK (2001a) *Cardiopulmonary Resuscitation. Guidance for Clinical Practice and Training in Hospitals*. Resuscitation Council UK, London.

Resuscitation Council UK (2001b) *Cardiopulmonary Resuscitation. Guidance for Clinical Practice and Training in Primary Care*. Resuscitation Council UK, London.

4 | Chain of Survival

INTRODUCTION

Effective resuscitation is dependent upon a number of different interventions happening within as short a time as possible. From the first moment when a bystander recognises and confirms a cardiac arrest right the way through until sophisticated management strategies are being considered in a specialist unit, the team's speed of response is of the utmost importance.

The members of the team are similar to a chain in that they are totally dependent on each other and if one link is not functioning, the chain breaks and team work fails. The 'Chain of Survival' therefore represents the combination of the individual components involved in the management of an emergency.

This idea of linking the basic resuscitation of first responders to the advanced life support may be seen as common sense. However, a great deal of time and money has been spent seeking to improve all aspects of the system and how those involved work together (Cummins *et al.* 1991).

AIMS

This chapter describes the development of the 'Chain of Survival' concept, its implementation and its relevance to current resuscitation practice.

LEARNING OUTCOMES

At the end of the chapter the reader will be able to:

❑ describe the *links* in the Chain of Survival;
❑ understand the *rationale* for developing the Chain of Survival;

❏ describe how the Chain of Survival *operates in both community and hospital settings.*

The four links in the Chain of Survival are shown in Figure 4.1.

DEVELOPMENT OF THE CHAIN OF SURVIVAL

The concept of the Chain of Survival has not changed significantly since it was first described even though individual components such as basic life support (BLS) and defibrillation have been refined and redirected.

The need to link the efforts of those responding to an emergency was described as far back as the 1960s. Its genesis was based on the pre-hospital setting to deal with the problem of sudden cardiac death (SCD) in the community. Peter Safar recognised the need to link basic cardiopulmonary resuscitation (CPR), whose aim was to 'buy time', to advanced life support (ALS), whose aim was to restore spontaneous circulation (Newman 1998). This message was developed by Mary Newman of the Citizen Foundation who introduced the Chain of Survival metaphor in 1987 (Newman 1989). By the mid-1980s the importance of early defibrillation had been established and as such became a component of the chain in its own right.

The first Chain of Survival was published in 1989 and had only three links which were:

• early access;
• early cardiopulmonary resuscitation;
• early defibrillation.

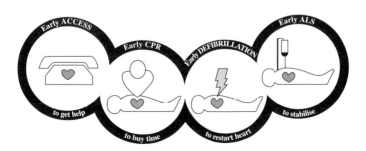

Fig. 4.1 Four links in the Chain of Survival.

Within a year the fourth link, that of early ALS, had been added (Newman 1989).

IMPLEMENTATION OF THE CHAIN OF SURVIVAL

Early access

The call to summon expert help and emergency equipment will either be a 999 call in the UK community setting or a cardiac arrest or 'crash' call in hospital. This will ensure that advanced airway/breathing equipment, a defibrillator and emergency drugs can be dispatched at the earliest opportunity.

Telephoning for assistance relies on the first rescuer assessing the casualty, accurately recognising the arrested state and then responding by summoning help.

Early access will not be achieved if the rescuer:

- chooses not to approach the casualty – real or perceived risks;
- fails to recognise cardiac arrest – inadequate training;
- does not know the number to phone – inadequate training.

Early CPR

Chest compressions achieve only 25–30% of normal cardiac output (Resuscitation Council UK 2000). Thus CPR delivers considerably less oxygen to vital organs than they normally receive so it cannot prevent organ damage over an extended period of time. This reinforces the need for early access to expert help in both the hospital and community settings.

The options open to the rescuer with regard to *how* to commence CPR will vary depending on the availability of equipment and expert assistance.

The purpose of CPR is to effectively perfuse the body's vital organs such as the heart and brain during the period of absent circulation. It will rarely restore spontaneous circulation on its own, which is why the next link in the chain is defibrillation.

Early defibrillation

Cardiopulmonary resuscitation is a means of 'buying time' for all casualties prior to the arrival of the defibrillator. However, if the defibrillator is immediately available, for example in a coronary care unit or ambulance, it should be used without delay. Approximately 30% of in-hospital arrests (Gwinnutt *et al.* 2000) and 80% of those out of hospital (Eisenberg & Mengert 2001) have shockable rhythms as their first recorded rhythms (see Chapter 9 for further details).

Early ALS

Many more lives have been saved by the application of the first three links of the Chain of Survival but effective and timely advanced life support will influence not only survival but also the quality of life. The interventions undertaken by a hospital cardiac arrest team or paramedics in the out-of-hospital setting will include intubation to protect the airway, securing intravenous access and administering cardiac arrest drugs. Whilst this is happening it is also essential to assess the casualty's clinical history for potentially reversible causes and ensure that CPR remains effective.

DEBATE SURROUNDING THE CHAIN OF SURVIVAL

'Phone First' or 'Phone Fast'

The question of whether the *lone rescuer* should initiate CPR or should first phone for help proved difficult to answer. If defibrillation is of such importance then access to help should come first. The counterargument ran that CPR provided oxygenation to the brain and may actually restore spontaneous circulation in some cases.

The Resuscitation Council UK (2000) guidelines recommend that the lone rescuer checks the casualty for breathing and signs of life and if these are absent, phones for help. The rescuer should then return to the casualty to carry out CPR until help arrives. Obviously if two or more rescuers are present, one can get expert help while the other commences resuscitation.

Exceptions to the 'Phone First' principle

The rationale for the recommendation to phone first was based on the likelihood of the rhythm being suitable for defibrillation in SCD.

Table 4.1 Arrests when one minute of CPR should be completed first.

Cause of arrest	Primary system involved
Submersion/near drowning	Airway/breathing
Arrest associated with trauma	Airway
Drug overdose	Respiratory depression
Children (who are not at risk of arrhythmias)	Airway/breathing

Casualties suffering from arrests that are not cardiac in origin will gain greater benefit from the completion of one minute of CPR to restore oxygenation, which in turn may bring the casualty back to life if it corrects the cause of the collapse.

Other examples of cardiac arrest, where the aetiology of the arrest is not primarily cardiac but is caused by failure in a different system, include the following:

- airway obstruction;
- respiratory failure;
- critical reduction in perfusion.

Paediatric cardiac arrests are more likely to be due to an airway/breathing problem leading to hypoxia. Immediate CPR to restore oxygen delivery would obviously be of greater value in this instance than a phone call for a defibrillator. It is estimated that paediatric arrests will present in shockable rhythms in approximately 10% of cases (Young & Siedel 1999) compared to 80% for adults (Eisenberg & Mengert 2001).

The situations in Table 4.1 are examples of when the lone rescuer should initially complete a full minute of CPR before leaving the casualty to phone for help.

HOW THE CHAIN OF SURVIVAL FUNCTIONS IN PRACTICE
This can be divided into pre-hospital and in-hospital settings.

The pre-hospital setting
There is continuing evidence supporting the importance of the chain working as a single unit rather than as separate entities. Researchers have clearly demonstrated that survival is severely diminished if a single link fails (Cummins *et al.* 1991).

Table 4.2 Effects of minimal delay.

Collapse to CPR	Collapse to defibrillation	
	<10 mins	>10 mins
<5 mins	37% survival	7% survival
>5 mins	20% survival	0% survival

How the chain may break

- Access – this may be delayed if the casualty is in an unsafe environment, is not found or if bystanders are either unwilling or lacking confidence to get involved.
- CPR – a lay person finding a casualty may phone for help very rapidly but then fail to provide effective CPR. Survival to discharge from out-of-hospital arrest doubles if CPR is started within four minutes (Larsen *et al.* 1993). Effective CPR is associated with a greater incidence of the first recorded rhythm being VF (Dowie *et al.* 2003).
- Defibrillation – even if a rapid phone call for help and bystander CPR do occur immediately, defibrillation may be delayed by a number of factors such as traffic and distance.

The success of the chain in the pre-hospital setting is demonstrated in examples where limited equipment is available, such as on aeroplanes (Page *et al.* 2000), railway stations (Davies 2002), in GP surgeries (Colquhoun 2002) and in Las Vegas casinos (Valenzuela *et al.* 2000). In all these settings the time from collapse to being found was short (early access), CPR was started promptly (early CPR) and they are all settings where shock advisory defibrillators were provided (early defibrillation).

Compared to the first three links, the introduction of drugs has had only limited impact (Mitchell *et al.* 2000).

Table 4.2 illustrates that where either early CPR or early defibrillation occurs, the survival is considerably less than if both occur with minimal delay (Cummins *et al.* 1985).

The ideal provision for out-of-hospital arrests includes:

- large percentage of the population know how to summon emergency help;

- high proportion of the public trained to recognise and respond to cardiac arrest;
- public access defibrillators and first responder schemes in place;
- rapid response from emergency medical services.

The in-hospital setting

When an inpatient has a cardiac arrest, their chances of surviving to discharge from hospital are approximately 1 in 7 (Gwinnutt *et al.* 2000).

In the hospital environment early access and early CPR should be achieved by appropriate staff training. In addition to this, many nurses and doctors will be available to defibrillate the casualty and provide ALS. At first glance, the Chain of Survival looks very strong so it is of concern that the overall in-hospital survival is only 17%.

Underlying factors for this survival rate might include the following.

- The degree of illness (co-morbidity) present in the in-hospital population. Compared to the general population, this group is more likely to be suffering from chronic disease. It has been shown that the greater the degree of chronic disease, the lower the chances of survival from cardiac arrest (Ambury *et al.* 2000).
- The first presenting cardiac rhythm, which is likely to be non-shockable. These cardiac arrest rhythms have lower survival rates than VF/VT arrests and are the presenting rhythm in two-thirds of in-hospital arrests (Gwinnutt *et al.* 2000).
- The patient is very likely to deteriorate either gradually or dramatically over a period of time. At the end of this period of inadequate ventilation or circulatory failure, the patient will be suffering some degree of hypoxia and multiorgan failure. Cardiac arrest in this instance will be more difficult to reverse.

The concept of the Chain of Survival has demonstrated that each link on its own has limited benefit unless all the links in the chain are present. When dealing with the sick or deteriorating in-hospital patient, it could be considered that there is a

'Chain of Responsibility'. When a critical incident occurs it is rarely found to be the fault of one individual but is more commonly proved to be a failure in the system (DoH 1998). Evidence of the failure of a system includes such examples as:

- deteriorating clinical signs not recorded;
- signs recorded but their importance not understood;
- signs recorded and understood but not reported;
- signs reported but not acted upon with necessary haste;
- acted on with sufficient haste but by insufficiently experienced personnel.

It is worth considering which of the examples above are the responsibility of the nurse looking after the patient. The first four examples are the nurse's direct responsibility, not that of the attending medical staff. It is certainly possible for the nurse to influence, if not ensure that expert help of the required seniority is summoned to the deteriorating patient.

Systems are now being routinely used in hospital settings to more rigorously monitor high-risk patients to recognise signs of deterioration and to increase speed of response from expert help, with the aim of preventing unnecessary cardiac arrests occurring (see Chapter 2).

REVIEW OF LEARNING

❏ The Chain of Survival has four components which are:
   - early access
   - early recognition
   - early defibrillation
   - early advanced life support.
❏ The aim is to link essential interventions with optimising survival.
❏ Early access stresses the importance of summoning help as the first priority.
❏ Early CPR 'buys time' prior to the arrival of advanced life support.
❏ Early defibrillation is the most important advanced intervention.

❏ Early advanced life support has the aims of restoring spontaneous circulation and stabilising the casualty post arrest.

❏ There are certain circumstances where the lone rescuer should perform CPR before telephoning for help.

❏ Out-of-hospital settings have dramatically improved access to defibrillation.

❏ The aim of a potential fifth link in the Chain of Survival is cardiac arrest prevention.

❏ In the out-of-hospital setting the priority is to improve early recognition of and response to acute myocardial infarction.

❏ In hospital the emphasis is on recognising patients at risk and responding quickly and effectively to prevent arrests occurring.

CONCLUSION

The Chain of Survival concept has always sought to promote the importance of reacting with speed to a cardiac arrest. The essential components rely on one another. If a single link is broken, the chain ceases to function. Today there is greater emphasis on the prevention of cardiac arrest because it has been so difficult to significantly improve arrest survival.

REFERENCES

Ambury, P., King, B. & Bannerjee, M. (2000) Does concurrent or previous illness accurately predict cardiac arrest survival? *Resuscitation* **47**, 267–71.

Colquhoun, M.C. (2002) Defibrillation by general practitioners. *Resuscitation* **52**, 143–8.

Cummins, R.O., Eisenberg, M.S., Hallstrom, A.P. & Litwin, P.E. (1985) Survival from out-of-hospital cardiac arrest with early initiation of cardiopulmonary resuscitation. *American Journal of Emergency Medicine* **3**, 114–19.

Cummins, R., Ornato, J., Thies, W. & Pepe, P. (1991) Improving survival from cardiac arrest: the chain of survival concept. *Circulation* **83**, 1832–47.

Davies, C.S. (2002) Defibrillators in public places: the introduction of a national scheme for public access defibrillation in England. *Resuscitation* **52**, 13–21.

Department of Health (1998) *Why Mothers Die. Report of Confidential Enquiries into Maternal Deaths in the United Kingdom 1994–1996.* Department of Health, London.

Dowie, R., Campbell, H., Donohoe, R. & Clarke, P. (2003) 'Event tree' analysis of out of hospital cardiac arrest data: confirming the importance of bystander CPR. *Resuscitation* **56**, 173–81.

Eisenberg, M.S. & Mengert, T.J. (2001) Cardiac resuscitation. *New England Journal of Medicine* **344** (17), 1304–13.

Gwinnutt, C.L., Columb, M. & Harris, R. (2000) Outcome after cardiac arrest in hospitals: effect of 1997 guidelines. *Resuscitation* **47**, 125–35.

Larsen, M.P., Eisenberg, M.S., Cummins, R.O. & Hallstrom, A.P. (1993) Predicting survival from out-of-hospital cardiac arrest: a graphic model. *Annals of Emergency Medicine* **22**, 1652–8.

Mitchell, R.G., Guly, U.M., Rainer, T.H. & Robertson, C.E. (2000) Paramedic activities, drug administration and survival from out-of-hospital cardiac arrest. *Resuscitation* **43**, 95–100.

Newman, M. (1989) Chain of survival concept takes hold. *Journal of Emergency Medical Services* **14** (8), 11–13.

Newman, M. (1998) Chain of survival revisited. *Journal of Emergency Medical Services* **23** (5), 47–56.

Page, R.L., Joglar, J.A. & Kowal, R.C. (2000) Use of advisory external defibrillators by a United States airline. *New England Journal of Medicine* **343**, 1210–16.

Resuscitation Council UK (2000) *Advanced Life Support Course Provider Manual*, 4th edn. Resuscitation Council UK, London.

Valenzuela, T.D., Roe, D., Nichol, G., Clark, L.L., Spaite, D.W. & Hardman, R.G. (2000) Outcome of rapid defibrillation by security officers after cardiac arrest in casinos. *New England Journal of Medicine* **343**, 1242–7.

Young, K.D. & Siedel, J.S. (1999) Paediatric cardiopulmonary resuscitation – a collective review. *Annals of Emergency Medicine* **33**, 195–205.

Section 3

Basic Life Support

5 | Basic Life Support Algorithm

INTRODUCTION

Basic life support (BLS) is employed in cardiorespiratory arrest and includes assessment of the collapsed person, maintaining airway patency, delivering expired air ventilation and external chest compressions (Resuscitation Council UK 2000a). It acts to support ventilation until the causes of arrest can be ascertained and, where possible, treated with defibrillation and drugs. Any delay in the administration of such life-preserving actions can result in permanent cerebral damage and therefore BLS must be initiated, following the recommended sequence of actions, as soon as a cardiac arrest is confirmed.

AIMS

This chapter presents the principles of basic life support (BLS).

LEARNING OUTCOMES

At the end of the chapter the reader should be able to:

❑ identify the *safety issues* associated with BLS;
❑ describe the *sequence of actions* undertaken in BLS;
❑ describe the *techniques* of BLS delivery;
❑ discuss the *differences between lay person and in-hospital BLS*;
❑ outline the approach to *initiating treatment with two rescuers*;
❑ discuss the *management of choking adults*;
❑ describe the sequence of actions undertaken in *using the recovery position*;
❑ outline the recommendations and developments in the *use of the automated external defibrillators* in BLS.

ADULT BASIC LIFE SUPPORT GUIDELINES

Updated resuscitation guidelines published in 2000 were based on the 'best evidence' base at the time and will no doubt continue to evolve as the availability of research knowledge in the field increases (American Heart Association (AHA) and International Liaison Committee on Resuscitation (ILCOR) 2000). The guidelines sought to develop a more streamlined approach to resuscitation, which differentiates between the health professional, often resuscitating in the hospital environment, and the out-of-hospital rescue.

SAFETY: REDUCING RISKS IN RESUSCITATION

Prior to entering the scene of a possible arrest, the rescuer should consider the following.

- Environment – the rescuer should review all possible hazards which in an out-of-hospital arrest might present as falling debris, traffic, electricity or water. In the hospital environmental hazards can include fluid spillage and equipment.
- Infection – the possible transmission of infection from a casualty or patient must be considered. There have been 15 documented cases of transfer in resuscitation and only three reported cases of HIV infection have occurred, resulting from deep needlestick injuries and heavy contamination of excoriated hands (Resuscitation Council UK 2000b). Careful use and disposal of needles are therefore required.
- Manual handling – safe handling techniques should be practised at all times, ensuring good posture during BLS and safe handling of the casualty (Resuscitation Council UK 2001).

OUT-OF-HOSPITAL RESUSCITATION

In out-of-hospital resuscitation, the casualty is often attended without the aid of any resuscitation equipment, such as airway adjuncts. The suggested algorithm includes assessment of safety, responsiveness, airway and breathing. If breathing is absent, the rescuer should call for help and then proceed to deliver breaths and check for circulation.

Checking for responsiveness

In the collapsed casualty, this requires a gentle shake of the casualty's shoulders whilst shouting into each ear, 'Are you all right?'.

If the casualty responds verbally or by moving:

- leave the casualty where they are, provided this is a safe environment;
- keep checking the casualty for a verbal response or movement;
- ensure dignity is maintained.

If the casualty does not respond:

- shout for immediate assistance;
- continue with your assessment, which might require moving the casualty on to their back to gain access to the airway and pulse.

Opening and clearing the airway

This manoeuvre reduces the risk of airway obstruction in the unconscious or unresponsive casualty. The procedure allows lifting of the jaw, moving the tongue away from the throat.

Head tilt/chin lift

- Open the casualty's airway with a head tilt/chin lift (see Figure 5.1).
- Place one of your hands on the casualty's forehead.
- Remove any visible debris from the mouth with your finger, but leave well-fitting dentures in place.
- With the tips of the index and middle fingers of your other hand on the hard palate (the bony prominence of the chin) lift the chin to open the airway.
- In suspected cervical spine injuries, care must be used when opening the airway, with the jaw thrust being preferred (see Figure 5.2).

Jaw thrust

- You should place both hands on either side of the casualty's head, whilst resting your elbows on the surface behind.
- The angle of the jaw beneath the ear is held and lifted, without tilting the head.
- The lower lip can be moved down if the lips are closed.

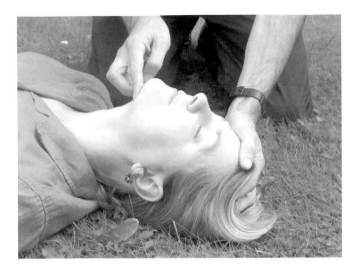

Fig. 5.1 Head tilt/chin lift.

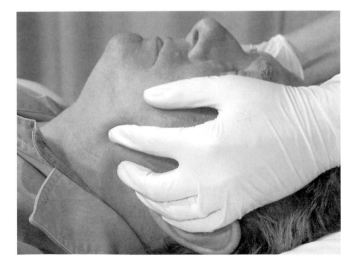

Fig. 5.2 Jaw thrust.

Look, listen and feel for breathing

Bringing the side of your face above that of the casualty, you should:

- look for signs of chest movement;
- listen for breath sounds;
- feel for breath on the side of your face.

This manoeuvre should be completed in no more than 10 seconds (see Figure 5.3).

If the casualty is breathing normally:

- employ the recovery position (see page 82 for a fuller explanation of this);
- continue to check for breathing signs, using the look, listen and feel manoeuvre;
- send someone else to summon help if you can, and ask them to report back to you;
- if alone, leave the casualty to summon help and return to the casualty as quickly as possible.

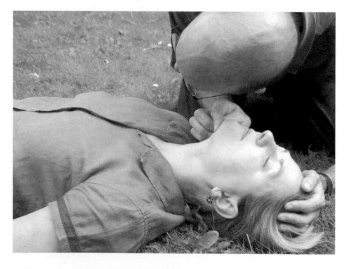

Fig. 5.3 Look, listen and feel for breathing.

If the breathing is absent or severely impaired with only occasional gasps seen:

- send someone else to call for emergency help if you can, and ask them to report back to you;
- if alone, leave the casualty to call for emergency help and return as quickly as possible to start rescue breathing.

In specific cases, where unconsciousness might be the result of breathing problems, the rescuer is advised to complete one minute of CPR. Such cases include:

- trauma;
- drowning/submersion;
- drug- or alcohol-induced unconsciousness;
- paediatric/children.

See Chapters 11, 13 and 14 for a fuller explanation of specific cases.

Breathing

Rescue breaths should be delivered slowly to avoid inflation of the stomach, which might lead to regurgitation of any stomach contents and possible pulmonary aspiration (Lawes & Baskett 1987).

Mouth-to-mouth breathing

- Ensure the airway is open (head tilt/chin lift).
- Ensuring the casualty is on their back, give two slow rescue breaths.
- The nose should be occluded by pinching the nostrils between the index finger and thumb of the hand you have on the casualty's forehead.
- The mouth must be open whilst a head tilt/chin lift is maintained.
- You should take a deep breath and place your mouth over the casualty's, ensuring a good seal.
- Exhale slowly, over two seconds.
- You need to observe the chest rise and fall, which gives a measure of the effectiveness of rescue breathing.
- A further deep breath should be taken and a second breath delivered.

- If rescue breathing is not effective, try repositioning the head tilt/chin lift and check for obstructions in the casualty's mouth.
- You can make up to five attempts to deliver two effective breaths.
- If you are unable to secure effective breathing, then proceed to assess for signs of circulation.
- Exhalation can be aided through opening the casualty's mouth at the appropriate time.

Use of mouth barriers/airway adjuncts

Rescuers may have access to barrier devices, such as faceshields or airway adjuncts. The use of faceshields is recommended, especially when attempting resuscitation in unfamiliar environments, away from home (AHA & ILCOR 2000). The dearth of research reviewing the effectiveness of faceshields results in a lack of evidence to support their use by healthcare professionals, for whom the use of masks is recommended when available (Simmons *et al.* 1995).

Use of a mouth mask

- The mask should be placed on the casualty's face, following the manufacturer's instructions.
- The seal of the mask on the face should be ensured by placing your thumbs and fingers around the lower portion of the mask and jaw (as in Chapter 7).
- Slow breaths are delivered through the mask non-return valve.
- Chest movements should be observed.

Assess for signs of circulation

If the rescuer is a lay person they should assess the casualty for signs of circulation and not be expected to undertake a carotid or femoral pulse check, though the healthcare professional should undertake this procedure as well.

- Look, listen and feel for any signs of life, such as breathing, coughing and movement.

- Assess the carotid pulse, if trained to do so.
- Maintain the head tilt with one hand on the casualty's forehead throughout the assessment.
- Using the index finger and middle finger of your free hand, trace down the trachea of the casualty and slide across to palpate the pulse between the trachea and sternocleidomastoid muscle, at the side of the neck.
- Apply gentle pressure over the carotid pulse for up to ten seconds.

If circulation is present
- Continue your rescue breathing.
- Recheck for signs of circulation every minute.
- If breathing recommences, place the casualty in the recovery position (see page 82).

If circulation is not present
- You should commence chest compressions.
- Locate the lower margin of the casualty's ribs with your index and middle fingers.
- Trace along the lower rib to the xiphoid, where the two ribs join the sternum.
- Place your two fingers on the sternum and bring the heel of your other hand down the sternum to touch your index finger.
- Take your other hand and place the heel on top of the hand already in position.
- Interlock the fingers of both hands to avoid compression of the ribs.
- You should ensure your own safe positioning, with knees apart, shoulders above the point of compression and elbows straight.
- Compressions must be delivered with an even movement, between 4 and 5 cm in depth.
- Release the chest, allowing it to rise, whilst maintaining hand contact and positioning over the point of compression.
- Repeat chest compressions at the rate of 100 compressions per minute.

Rescue breathing and compression

If acting as a single rescuer, you will need to perform these manoeuvres alone. If working in a team of rescuers, you should adopt roles in delivering rescue breathing or chest compressions, rotating roles as necessary.

- Cycles of two breaths followed by 15 compressions should be maintained as the most effective ratio (Wik & Steen 1996).
- Cycles should not be interrupted unless the casualty shows signs of life, such as breathing or moving.
- Efforts must be continued until emergency help arrives or until you are unable to maintain them.

IN-HOSPITAL BASIC LIFE SUPPORT

This approach is emphasised for use by healthcare professionals attending the collapsed patient in the hospital setting. The provision of resuscitation equipment within the hospital and some pre-hospital settings, such as ambulance paramedics, necessitates the modification of BLS guidelines. The initial management of arrest in these circumstances is depicted in the in-hospital basic life support algorithm (see Figure 5. 4).

Patient collapse

Once safety in the environment is established, the healthcare professional should call for help and perform the shake-and-shout procedure. Once colleagues are available to help, a number of actions can be undertaken in the initial phase of managing an arrest.

Breathing and pulse check

- You should observe for signs of breathing and for circulation.
- In some cases it is recommended that these checks are made simultaneously.

If the breathing and pulse are present:

- summon emergency medical support;
- start to administer oxygen;
- attach ECG monitoring leads and commence monitoring;
- secure venous access if this is not already in place.

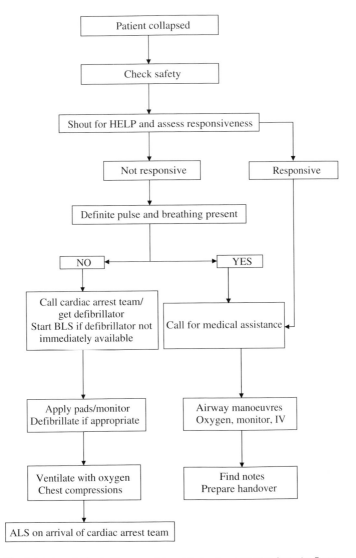

Fig. 5.4 In-hospital basic life support (reprinted with permission from the Resuscitation Council UK).

If breathing and pulse are absent members of the team should initiate the following.

- Summon the cardiac arrest team immediately using the local emergency number.
- Commence BLS.
- Ensure resuscitation equipment and the defibrillator are accessible at the patient's side.
- Support the airway and ventilation using available equipment, such as a pocket mask, oropharyngeal airway, LMA or bag-valve-mask (see Chapter 7 for further explanation of this equipment).
- Ensure oxygen is delivered at a tidal volume of 400–600 ml to reduce gastric inflation.
- Proceed in delivering two ventilations and 15 chest compressions until the patient is intubated with a secure cuffed tracheal tube or LMA.
- As a priority, the electrodes of either a manual or automated external defibrillator (AED) should be attached to the patient and used as necessary (see Chapter 9 for further explanation).
- Intravenous access should be secured, if not already available.
- You should prepare to hand over to the arriving cardiac arrest team, providing access to the patient's notes.
- If the patient's relatives or other patients are in the vicinity, ensure members of the nursing team are available to provide appropriate support.

Recovery position

The recovery position is vital in maintaining support of the airway, as it ensures the tongue is held in a forward position and it reduces the chance of inhalation of any expelled gastric contents (Resuscitation Council UK 2000a).

Whilst placing a casualty in the recovery position, make sure you maintain your own good posture and prevent injuries to yourself and the casualty.

- Make sure the environment is safe; check for potential hazards such as broken glass.

- Remove any hazards from the casualty, such as work tools or spectacles.
- Kneel next to the casualty.
- Ensure the casualty has straight legs and is lying on their back.
- Move the arm closest to you so that it is at right angles to the casualty's body, with the palm of the hand facing upwards.
- The other arm should be positioned across the chest, with the back of the hand placed next to the casualty's cheek. The hand should be held in this position.
- The leg furthest away from you should be bent at the knee, ensuring the foot is in contact with the ground.
- Pull on the leg, whilst maintaining hold of the hand on the cheek, to roll the casualty towards you onto their side.
- Move the upper leg to ensure it is at right angles to the casualty, supporting a stable position.
- Ensure the airway is open, tilting the head back if necessary and using the hand to support the positioning of the head (see Figures 5.5a–d and Box 5.1).

Box 5.1 Best practice – monitoring the casualty in the recovery position

Frequently check breathing rate and depth.

Observe the circulation to the lower arm that the casualty is lying on.

Turn the casualty onto their opposite side if they are required to remain in the recovery position for more than 30 minutes.

Preserve dignity throughout.

Choking

The Resuscitation Council UK guidelines (2000a) identify a three-stage approach to recognising and responding to the choking adult. These relate to the choking conscious casualty, the casualty who is conscious but deteriorating and finally the unconscious casualty.

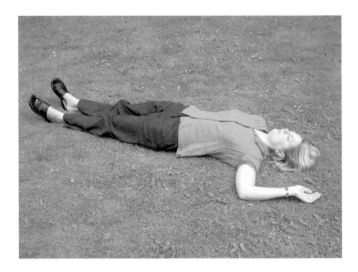

Fig. 5.5a Putting the patient in the recovery position.

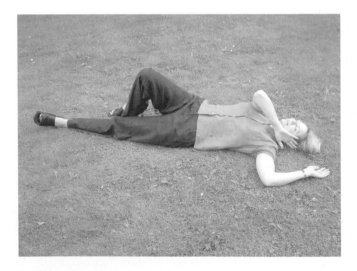

Fig. 5.5b Putting the patient in the recovery position.

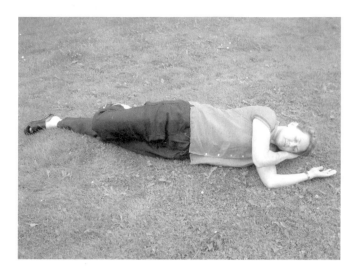

Fig. 5.5c Putting the patient in the recovery position.

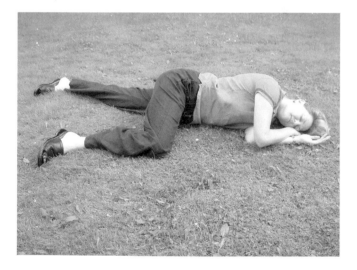

Fig. 5.5d The recovery position.

Conscious, breathing casualty

If the casualty appears to be choking but is conscious and coughing, no further action should be necessary other than to encourage continued coughing, observing for relief of the obstruction.

Casualty is deteriorating

If the casualty becomes tired, has been unable to relieve the obstruction or exhibits signs of cyanosis, such as blueness around the lips, perform the following manoeuvres.

- Commence back blows. Clear the mouth of any obvious obstruction. Stand to the side and slightly behind the casualty. Encourage the casualty to lean forwards, to support outward projection of any obstruction. Deliver up to five blows with the heel of your hand, between the scapulae (see Figure 5.6).
- If the obstruction persists, start abdominal thrusts. Stand behind the casualty, wrap your arms around the waist and ensure the casualty is leaning forwards. Make a fist with one hand and close the other hand on top of it. Position your hands below the xiphisternum. Pull your hands inwards and upwards (see Figure 5.7). Check to see if the obstruction has cleared.
- Up to five back blows and five abdominal thrusts can be alternated until the obstruction is cleared.

Casualty collapses and is unconscious

If back blows and abdominal thrusts fail and the casualty becomes unconscious, a sequence of life support is recommended, as in the managing of the choking adult algorithm (Resuscitation Council UK 2000a) (see Figure 5.8). If there is no evidence of breathing then ventilation should be attempted. Where this fails, chest compressions should be maintained. If it is possible to ventilate the casualty, circulation should be checked. If this is absent then start BLS.

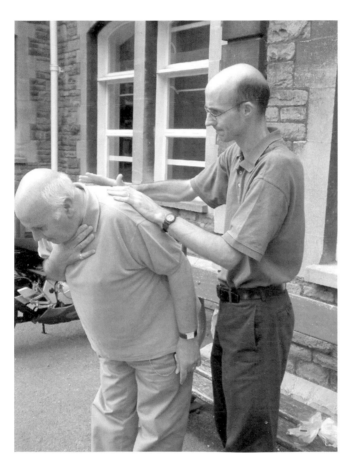

Fig. 5.6 Back blows.

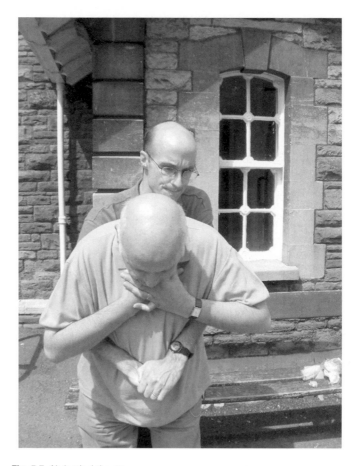

Fig. 5.7 Abdominal thrusts.

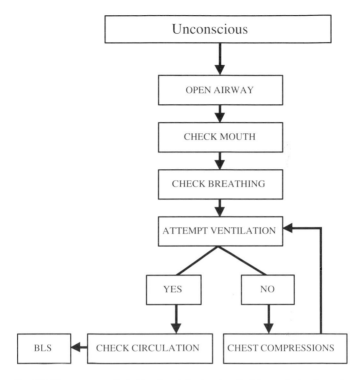

Fig. 5.8 Management of choking in adults (reprinted with permission from the Resuscitation Council UK).

REVIEW OF LEARNING

❏ Basic life support includes: assessing safety of the environment, checking response, opening and clearing the airway, checking breathing, delivering breaths if needed, checking for circulation and delivering chest compressions if required.
❏ In the hospital setting defibrillators may be employed.
❏ It is important to call for emergency help after establishing the presence or absence of breathing.
❏ The recovery position is vital in maintaining the support of the airway in the collapsed casualty.

Case study

Mr Coughlin, a 73 year old, is visiting his son in his new home. He has been digging the garden and comes into the house clutching his chest. He collapses to the floor and his wife and son are unable to rouse him. The son rushes across the street to find help. You are one of two rescuers who attend the house. You are both student nurses who have recently had BLS training. **What should you do?**

Before reading on, make a list of your actions.

Firstly you should check that the environment is safe to enter, then assess the casualty for a response. Next you should open and clear the airway and check for the presence of breathing and circulation. This reveals that Mr Coughlin is unresponsive and not breathing. You order the son to contact the emergency services. There are no signs of life and on checking the pulse, you find this is also absent. Your friend explains to Mr Coughlin's wife and son about the need to perform BLS.

In line with guidelines, you commence BLS as per two-person recommendations. One of you delivers the breaths and the other chest compressions at a ratio of 2:15.

You rotate roles to reduce exhaustion. After 20 minutes the emergency services arrive and are able to insert an oropharyngeal airway, administer oxygen via a mask and apply defibrillator pads whilst you continue BLS. This unfortunately reveals that Mr Coughlin has no cardiac output and an asystolic rhythm is seen on the monitor screen.

CONCLUSION

The guidelines for BLS are designed to aid recall and support effective resuscitation and all healthcare professionals should be familiar with the most up-to-date guidelines. Accessing the *Resuscitation* journal and Resuscitation Council UK and European Resuscitation Council websites (www.resus.org.uk and www.erc.edu) will ensure that practice remains updated.

REFERENCES

American Heart Association and International Liaison Committee on Resuscitation (2000) Part 3. Adult basic life support. *Resuscitation* **46**, 29–71.

Lawes, E. & Baskett, P. (1987) Pulmonary aspiration during unsuccessful cardiopulmonary resuscitation: a comparison between the bag valve mask and laryngeal mask airway resuscitation. *Intensive Care Medicine* **13**, 370–82.

Resuscitation Council UK (2000a) *Resuscitation Guidelines*. Resuscitation Council UK, London.

Resuscitation Council UK (2000b) *Advanced Life Support Course Provider Manual*, 4th edn. Resuscitation Council UK, London.

Resuscitation Council UK (2001) *Guidance on Safe Handling*. Resuscitation Council UK, London.

Simmons, M., Deano, D., Moon, L., Peters, K. & Cavanaugh, S. (1995) Bench evaluation: three face shield CPR barrier devices. *Respiratory Care* **40**, 618–23.

Wik, L. & Steen, P. (1996) The ventilation–compression ratio influences the effectiveness of two-rescuer advanced cardiac life support on a manikin. *Resuscitation* **31**, 113–19.

Section 4

Advanced Life Support

6 | The Universal Advanced Life Support Algorithm

INTRODUCTION

Advanced life support is an essential link in the Chain of Survival. The universal algorithm provides a sequence of actions for the management of all people who appear in cardiac arrest – unconscious, unresponsive, without signs of life. Cardiac arrest may present as a *shockable* rhythm, such as ventricular fibrillation or pulseless ventricular tachycardia (VF/VT), or a *non-shockable* rhythm such as asystole or pulseless electrical activity (PEA). Attempts at defibrillation will be necessary in cases of VF/VT. Other actions, including chest compressions, airway management and ventilation, venous access, drug administration and correction of possible causes, are common to both these rhythms. The algorithm is applicable universally but cardiac arrest may occur in special circumstances, for example hypothermia, drug overdose and electrical injury. Additional interventions may be necessary, as discussed in Chapter 13.

The universal algorithm was based on collaborative research from resuscitation experts around the world. All information in this chapter is drawn from the references noted at the end.

AIMS

This chapter expands on each step of the advanced life support (ALS) universal treatment algorithm (see Figure 6.1).

LEARNING OUTCOMES

At the end of the chapter the reader should be able to:

❑ describe the *sequence of actions* in the universal algorithm;
❑ understand the management of *patients in a 'shockable' rhythm* (VF/VT);
❑ understand the management of *patients in a 'non-shockable' rhythm* (PEA, asystole).

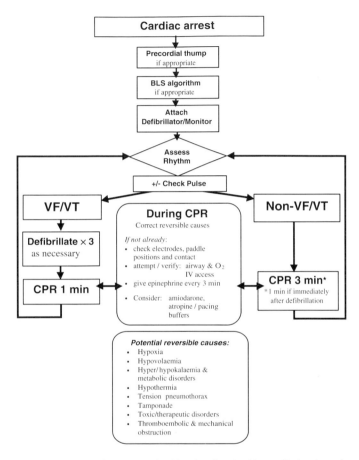

Fig. 6.1 Advanced life support algorithm (reprinted with permission from the Resuscitation Council UK).

SHOCKABLE RHYTHMS: VENTRICULAR FIBRILLATION AND PULSELESS VENTRICULAR TACHYCARDIA

The majority of people who collapse from a cardiac arrest in the community are in VF and are those most likely to survive (AHA & ILCOR 2000). Whatever the setting, hospital, community or home, successful resuscitation depends on early defibrillation (White *et al.* 1996). The chance of successful defibrillation declines with each minute that VF persists. While effective basic life support (BLS) slows the irreversible damage, it cannot stop it. The patient's rhythm needs to be assessed as soon as possible, preferably with monitoring electrodes from an automatic or manual defibrillator. A dedicated electrocardiogram (ECG) monitor may also be used (see Chapter 8). The first shock should be delivered as soon as possible if the rhythm is VF/VT. (For further information about this arrhythmia see Chapter 8.) If a monitor is not readily available, BLS should be continued until a defibrillator arrives.

The discussion that follows provides a step-by-step account of the ALS algorithm (see Figure 6.1) and the activities that must be performed for patients in either VF/VT or PEA cardiac arrest, once cardiac arrest is confirmed (Resuscitation Council UK 2000a).

Precordial thump
- A single precordial thump is an acceptable and possibly helpful action in a witnessed or monitored arrest when a defibrillator is not immediately available (Resuscitation Council UK 2000c).
- Give a sharp blow with a closed fist on the patient's sternum. If this is done within 30 seconds after the arrest, it may be enough to successfully convert the patient's heart back to a perfusing rhythm.
- Reassess circulation after delivery of a precordial thump.

Defibrillating the patient
- Three shocks – give up to three shocks initially with energies of 200 J, 200 J, 360 J (or their biphasic equivalent). These shocks should be delivered one after the other without a delay. If all three shocks are necessary, try to give them in less than one minute.
- Between shocks – when more than one shock is required, the electrodes (AED) or paddles (manual defibrillator) should be left on the patient's chest while the defibrillator is recharging.

Be aware of the possibility of spurious asystole, a short delay after delivering a shock before the monitor recovers the display of the heart rhythm. Always reassess the rhythm just before delivering the shock (Bradbury *et al.* 2000). See also Chapter 9.

- Electrical and myocardial stunning – after defibrillation there is often a brief delay before the ECG settles and the rhythm can be interpreted. Successful defibrillation may be followed by a few seconds of asystole, referred to as electrical stunning (Resuscitation Council UK 2000b). Also, even if the rhythm is one that is normally compatible with a pulse, there may be a few seconds of impaired myocardial contractility. This is called myocardial stunning and results in a pulse that is weak and difficult to palpate. It is essential not to make a diagnosis of PEA or asystole too soon as defibrillation may have been successful. The algorithm indicates doing one minute of CPR before reassessing the rhythm and rechecking the pulse. It is important not to give any drugs during this minute. They could be harmful if a perfusing rhythm is present (AHA & ILCOR 2000).

During CPR

- Chest compressions – VF may persist after the delivery of three shocks. Early defibrillation is still the best way to restore a perfusing rhythm but it is important to maintain cerebral and myocardial viability. Therefore, one minute of CPR with a compression-to-ventilation ratio of 15:2 should be started without delay (AHA & ILCOR 2000).

- Airway and ventilation – it will be impossible to restart the heart without adequate oxygenation. Secure the patient's airway and deliver the highest possible concentration of oxygen. Tracheal intubation is the most reliable means to secure the airway, but a trained and experienced healthcare provider must perform this (Resuscitation Council UK 2000c). An LMA or Combitube may be inserted instead. Once the trachea has been intubated, chest compressions should be performed at a continuous rate of 100/min, stopping only for defibrillation, pulse checks or checking for a return of spontaneous circulation (AHA & ILCOR 2000). Ventilation should be continued at approximately 12 breaths/min. If an LMA has been inserted, attempt to perform continuous chest compressions, uninterrupted during ventilation. If this is not possible due to excessive gas leakage resulting in inadequate ventilation, use a 15:2 compression-to-ventilation ratio (see Chapter 5).

- Intravenous access – an intravenous line is essential for giving drugs and fluids. This can be achieved by central or peripheral venous access. Central veins are ideal because drugs can be delivered rapidly into the circulation. Cannulation of a peripheral vein is the procedure of choice because it is quicker, easier and safer.

- Drugs – drugs administered by the peripheral route must be followed by at least a 20 ml flush of 0.9% saline and if possible elevation of the extremity. Give epinephrine (adrenaline) 1 mg intravenously (Resuscitation Council UK 2000b). Pre-filled syringes like those described in Chapter 10 may be used.

- Amiodarone – amiodarone, an antiarrhythmic, can be considered following epinephrine in VF/VT that persists after the first three shocks (see Chapter 10). It can be given before the fourth shock as long as subsequent defibrillation is not delayed (AHA & ILCOR 2000).

Reassessing the rhythm
- Further defibrillation attempts – if the patient is still in VF after one minute of CPR, give up to three more shocks at 360 J (or biphasic equivalent), checking the monitor between shocks. Do not exceed one minute between the third and fourth shock, even if the airway or intravenous access is not secured (Resuscitation Council UK 2000c). If the patient has a restoration of a perfusing rhythm but then has a recurrence of VF/VT, defibrillation should start again at 200 J (or biphasic equivalent).

- Continuing the loop – the 'shockable' loop of the algorithm is continued with sequences of three shocks followed by one minute of CPR. Further attempts at securing the airway and establishing IV access are made if necessary. Continue to give epinephrine 1 mg every loop.

- Consider causes – it is important to treat any of the four Hs and four Ts (see Chapter 11). The number of times the loop is repeated depends on the clinical situation and the likelihood of a successful outcome. It is usually considered worthwhile continuing as long as the patient remains in VF/VT.

- Other issues – poor electrode or paddle contact will reduce the chances of successful defibrillation (Bradbury *et al.* 2000). Try a different defibrillator if one is available. The position of the paddles may also be changed to anteroposterior (one to the right of the sternum, the other between the shoulder blades as discussed in Chapter 9).

NON-SHOCKABLE RHYTHMS: PULSELESS ELECTRICAL ACTIVITY/ASYSTOLE

The outcome for 'non-shockable' rhythms is poor (AHA & ILCOR 2000). The team must rapidly consider and effectively treat the potential reversible causes. If PEA or asystole occurs immediately after a shock, it may be 'myocardial stunning' (see page 97). Continue CPR for one minute without giving any drugs. After one minute, re-check the rhythm and pulse. If PEA or aystole is still present, continue with a further two minutes of CPR and give the appropriate drugs.

Pulseless electrical activity (PEA)

- This condition is the presence of electrical activity normally associated with a cardiac output and the absence of a detectable pulse (see Chapters 8 and 11).
- Early identification and treatment will give the patient the best chance of survival (see later discussion). Continue resuscitation while identifying causes (Kloeck 1995).
- Follow the 'right loop' of the algorithm. CPR is started immediately and carried out for three minutes. Manage the airway and ventilation and initiate IV access. Epinephrine 1 mg is administered intravenously every three minutes. Atropine 3 mg IV may be given if the PEA is associated with bradycardia (<60/min) (Resuscitation Council UK 2000c).

Asystole
- Diagnose aystole correctly to ensure VF is not missed. Aystole can be confirmed by checking that leads are attached correctly and the rhythm is viewed through leads I or II. Increasing the gain on the monitor may also aid correct identification (for further detail refer to Chapter 8). If there is any doubt, follow the shockable side of the algorithm for VF (AHA & ILCOR 2000).
- Early identification and treatment will give the patient the best chance of survival (see later discussion). Continue resuscitation while identifying causes.
- Follow the 'right loop' of the algorithm. CPR is started immediately and carried out for three minutes. Manage the airway and ventilation and initiate IV access. Epinephrine 1 mg is administered intravenously every three minutes. Administer atropine 3 mg intravenously to give total blockade of the vagus nerve (Resuscitation Council UK 2000c).
- Check the ECG carefully for the presence of a P wave or slow ventricular activity. These rhythms may respond to cardiac pacing (AHA & ILCOR 2000).

During the treatment of PEA or asystole, the rhythm may change to VF/VT. Follow the shockable side of the algorithm if this happens.

POTENTIALLY REVERSIBLE CAUSES
The potentially reversible causes of cardiac arrest are divided into two groups to aid memory – four Hs and four Ts (see Chapter 11).

REVIEW OF LEARNING
- ❏ The universal algorithm provides a sequence of actions for the management of all people who appear in cardiac arrest, namely those who are unconscious, unresponsive, without signs of life.
- ❏ Cardiac arrest may present as a 'shockable' rhythm, such as ventricular fibrillation or pulseless ventricular tachycardia (VF/VT), or a 'non-shockable' rhythm, such as asystole or pulseless electrical activity (PEA).

❏ The chance of successful defibrillation declines with each minute that VF persists. The first shock should be delivered as soon as possible if the rhythm is VF/VT.

❏ The outcome for 'non-shockable' rhythms is poor. The team must rapidly consider and effectively treat the potentially reversible causes.

CONCLUSION

The universal algorithm provides a guide for the actions to take and decisions to make for all patients who appear to be in cardiac arrest. It is divided into shockable and non-shockable rhythms. All those involved in carrying out advanced life support should keep abreast of the most up-to-date guidelines, by regularly accessing the *Resuscitation* journal and Resuscitation Council UK and European Resuscitation Council websites (www.resus.org.uk and www.erc.edu/).

REFERENCES

American Heart Association and International Liaison Committee on Resuscitation (AHA & ILCOR) (2000) Part 6. Advanced cardiovascular life support. *Resuscitation* **46**, 140–57.

Bradbury, N., Hyde, D. & Nolan, J. (2000) Reliability of ECG monitoring with a gel pad/paddle combination after defibrillation. *Resuscitation* **44**, 203–6.

Kloeck, W.G. (1995) A practical approach to the aetiology of pulseless electrical activity: a simple 10-step training mnemonic. *Resuscitation* **30**, 157–9.

Resuscitation Council UK (2000a) *Resuscitation Guidelines*. Resuscitation Council UK, London.

Resuscitation Council UK (2000b) *Advanced Life Support Universal Algorithm*. Available online at: www.resus.org.uk

Resuscitation Council UK (2000c) *Advanced Life Support Course Provider Manual*, 4th edn. Resuscitation Council UK, London.

White, R., Asplin, B., Bugliosi, T. & Hankins, D. (1996) High discharge survival rate after out-of-hospital ventricular fibrillation with rapid defibrillation by police and paramedics. *Annals of Emergency Medicine* **28**, 480–5.

Section 5

Further Considerations of Resuscitation

7 | Management of the Airway and Breathing

INTRODUCTION

Airway management is an essential part of basic and advanced life support. In a patient who is breathing spontaneously, supplemental oxygen may prevent a cardiac or respiratory arrest. Any person in respiratory distress or cardiovascular crisis should also receive supplemental oxygen. During cardiac arrest it will be impossible to restart the heart without adequate oxygenation. Recognising airway and breathing problems promptly and responding with appropriate interventions will ensure hypoxic damage to vital organs is minimised.

AIMS

This chapter considers the management of airway and breathing in the compromised patient.

LEARNING OUTCOMES

At the end of the chapter the reader should be able to:

❑ discuss *potential causes* of airway obstruction;
❑ recognise airway problems using a *systematic assessment*;
❑ respond to airway and breathing problems with *appropriate interventions*;
❑ appreciate *advanced airway and breathing issues*.

REVIEW OF THE NORMAL AIRWAY

The airway is divided into the upper airway and lower airway. The upper airway comprises the nose, mouth and pharynx. The lower airway comprises the larynx, trachea and lungs. During normal breathing, oxygenated air enters the lungs through an open airway and oxygenates the blood. This is transported to the tissues providing the circulation is adequate. A lack of oxygen causes tissue hypoxia. Some organs are more sensitive to hypoxia. For example, if deprived of oxygen even for a short period of time, the brain is adversely affected. The patient may become agitated or confused and eventually their level of consciousness will deteriorate, leading to potentially irreversible or fatal brain damage.

Carbon dioxide is exhaled in normal breathing. An airway obstruction or breathing difficulty may result in the build-up of carbon dioxide in the blood (hypercarbia). The patient will appear drowsy or lethargic.

AIRWAY OBSTRUCTION

Airway obstruction may be either the result of or cause of loss of consciousness. The patient may have partial or complete obstruction and it may occur anywhere from the nose and mouth down to the bronchi (see Table 7.1). The tongue is the most common cause of airway obstruction in the unresponsive casualty (Baskett *et al.* 1996).

Table 7.1 Common causes of airway obstruction.

Level of obstruction		Potential causes
Upper airway	Mouth, nose, pharynx (often referred to nasopharynx, oropharynx and hypopharynx)	Most common – loss of pharyngeal muscle tone; vomit, blood, foreign body; epiglottis swelling; soft tissue oedema
Lower airway	Larynx	Oedema, laryngospasm (spasm of vocal cords); foreign body, trauma
	Trachea	Secretions or foreign body; swelling
	Lungs (the trachea branches into the right and left bronchi; lower passageways are called bronchioles)	Bronchospasm; pulmonary oedema; aspiration

Recognising an airway problem

The best way to recognise a partial or complete airway obstruction is by looking, listening and feeling (Baskett *et al.* 1996).

Look

- The patient who is able to verbalise clearly has an airway that is patent and not compromised at this point.
- An agitated and/or confused patient may be hypoxic.
- A lethargic patient may be hypercarbic.
- A cyanotic and pale patient is likely to be hypoxic. The skin may also be clammy or sweaty. Note that cyanosis is often a late sign and absence of cyanosis does not mean that the patient is adequately oxygenated.
- A patient showing signs of muscular retractions, who is making use of their accessory muscles or has shallow, laboured breathing has some degree of airway compromise.

Listen

- A patient whose respiration is quiet and effortless is breathing normally.
- Noisy breathing indicates partial airway obstruction (see Table 7.2).
- If there are no breath sounds, this indicates the absence of air entry that may be due to complete airway obstruction.

Table 7.2 Obstructive airway sounds.

Characteristic sounds	What they mean
Crowing	Laryngeal spasm or obstruction
Wheeze	An expiratory noise suggestive of lower airway obstruction
Stridor	An inspiratory noise suggestive of upper airway obstruction
Gurgling	Suggestive of liquid or semisolid foreign material in the main airways
Snoring	Indicates the pharynx is partially occluded by the tongue or palate

Feel
- A patient whose chest is moving equally and quietly, exhaling warm air, is breathing normally.
- If air cannot be felt but chest and abdominal movements are obvious, this is indicative of complete airway obstruction.

Basic airway opening techniques

Basic airway opening manoeuvres are simple techniques that can be performed anywhere and without the use of equipment. In most situations, the commonly used techniques of head tilt/chin lift and/or jaw thrust will be all that is required to relieve airway obstruction caused by the relaxation of soft tissues. These very basic manoeuvres have been described as part of basic life support (BLS) in Chapter 5.

- It is imperative that once a manoeuvre has been performed, it must not be assumed that it has been successful in opening the airway.
- Assessment should continue, using the look, listen and feel approach.
- If it is not possible to achieve a clear airway using either of these manoeuvres, it may be necessary to consider the use of suction or a simple airway adjunct.
- If there is evidence of trauma or any reason to suspect cervical spine injury, the jaw thrust is the airway opening technique of choice (American Heart Association (AHA) & International Liaison Committee on Resuscitation (ILCOR) 2000).

Oropharyngeal suctioning

The patient may have liquid (gastric contents, saliva, blood) present in the upper airway. This has the potential to cause airway obstruction or aspiration and therefore needs to be removed from the upper airway as quickly as possible.

There are a variety of suction devices available to assist in clearing the upper airway. The commonest device is a wide-bore rigid sucker (Yankauer), which is attached to a suction apparatus. Important points to remember are:

- the rescuer should always wear gloves when suctioning the patient;

107

• to perform oropharyngeal suctioning, the suction device should be carefully inserted into the patient's mouth. The tip of the suction device should be visible at all times to avoid stimulating a gag reflex.

Figure 7.1 illustrates a Yankauer sucker and suction unit.

AIRWAY ADJUNCTS

Airway adjuncts help improve and maintain an open and patent airway. Commonly used adjuncts include the oropharyngeal airway and nasopharyngeal airway. Both of these adjuncts can be used in the patient who is unconscious and has stopped breathing. In this situation the adjuncts help maintain airway patency during the use of ventilatory devices such as the pocket mask or bag-valve-mask system (AHA & ILCOR 2000). The unconscious patient who has stopped breathing may also benefit from the insertion of a device such as an LMA or Combitube, both of which offer a slightly more secure airway when personnel skilled in endotracheal intubation are not immediately available (Stone *et al.* 1998).

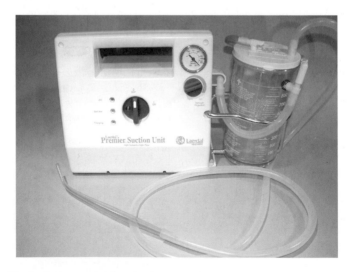

Fig. 7.1 Battery-operated suction device with Yankaeur suction catheter attached.

Pharyngeal airways

The oropharyngeal and nasopharyngeal airways are devices that help to prevent backward displacement of the tongue in an unconscious patient. It is important to note that a degree of head tilt, chin lift or jaw thrust will still be necessary when using an airway adjunct (AHA & ILCOR 2000). The patient who has an oropharyngeal or nasopharyngeal airway *in situ* but is breathing spontaneously will require supplemental oxygen via a delivery system (as described in Chapter 2). Failure to administer oxygen to seriously ill patients will compromise their chances of survival.

Oropharyngeal airway

For details on equipment design and indications for use, refer to Chapter 3.

Sizing
- Estimate the correct size by holding the airway vertically between the angle of the jaw and the incisors (as shown in Figure 7.2).
- An incorrectly sized airway, one that is too long or too short, may further obstruct the patient's airway or be ineffective.

Insertion technique (see Figure 7.3)
- Open the patient's mouth and ensure it is clear of any debris or foreign material.
- Insert the airway into the mouth in what initially appears to be the 'upside down' position until it is approximately halfway inserted.
- Rotate the airway 180° and continue to push it into place in the oral cavity. The reinforced section should sit firmly between the patient's teeth with the flange to the outside of the lips. If the patient does not have teeth, the reinforced section should rest between the gums.
- Assess the patient for airway and breathing, using the look, listen, feel sequence.

Nasopharyngeal airway

For details on equipment design and indications for use, refer to Chapter 3.

Sizing

- Sizes for this airway indicate the internal diameter in millimetres. As diameter size increases, so does the length.
- The following sizes are a guideline. However, common sense should be used when choosing the size.
    - —Large adult: 8.0–9.0
    - —Medium adult: 7.0–8.0
    - —Small adult: 6.0–7.0
- A tube that is too long may enter the oesophagus or may cause laryngospasm and vomiting.

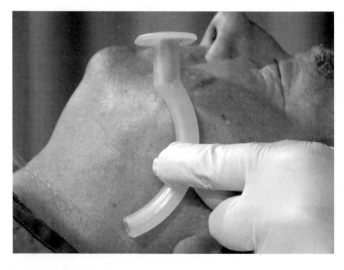

Fig. 7.2 Correct sizing of an oropharyngeal airway.

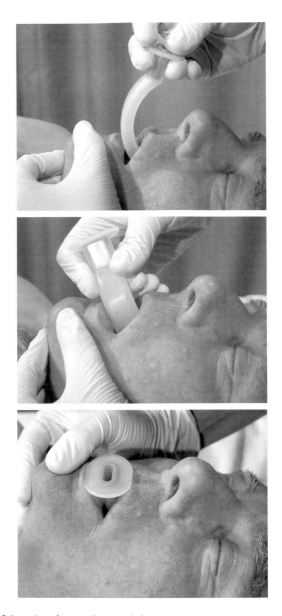

Fig. 7.3 Insertion of an oropharyngeal airway.

Insertion technique (see Figure 7.4)
- Check patency of the patient's nostrils. Generally the right nostril is preferred.
- Ensure that the airway is well lubricated with a water-soluble jelly. Some nasopharyngeal airways also require the insertion of a safety pin at the trumpet end to give extra protection against the airway slipping beyond the nostril.
- Insert the angular end into the patient's nostril and slide the airway along the floor of the nose by using a small twisting motion (in a patient who is supine, this is in a downward vertical direction).
- If there is any obstruction, try inserting the airway into the left nostril.
- Assess the patient for airway and breathing using the look, listen, feel sequence.
- Injury to the nasal mucosa may occur during insertion, leading to bleeding or problems when removing the airway. Always be prepared with suction to remove secretions or blood.

Laryngeal mask airway (LMA)

For details on equipment design and indications for use, refer to Chapter 3.

The LMA may be inserted almost immediately in the patient who has stopped breathing and become deeply unconscious.

There is some evidence to suggest that when a bag-valve device is used to ventilate the patient prior to insertion of the LMA, gastric regurgitation and aspiration are more likely to occur than if the LMA has been inserted immediately, without prior ventilation, as a first-line airway adjunct (Stone *et al.* 1998).

Once a ventilatory device such as a bag-valve has been attached to the LMA, it is important that high inflation pressures are not generated during ventilation as this increases the risk of gastric inflation and therefore potential regurgitation and aspiration.

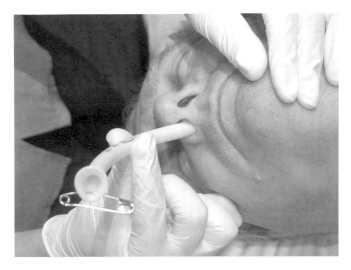

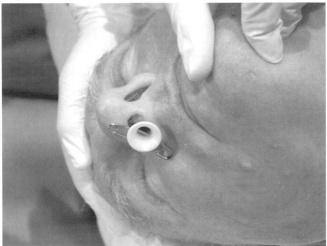

Fig. 7.4 Insertion of a nasopharyngeal airway.

Sizing
- The LMA is available in sizes suitable for neonates through to large adults.
- A size 4 or 5 is suitable for all but very small adults, who may be more suited to a size 3.

Insertion technique (see Figure 7.5)
- Check the cuff patency by inserting the appropriate amount of air (as shown in Table 7.3). Deflate the cuff and ensure the outer face of the cuff is lubricated.
- Position the patient supine with the head and neck aligned. Slightly flex the neck and extend the head unless there is suspicion of cervical spine injury.
- Hold the tube like a pen and introduce the cuff into the patient's mouth. Using the index finger to provide support at the tip of the cuff, advance it along the roof of the patient's mouth into the airway until it reaches the back of the throat.
- Take hold of the external part of the tube and, keeping it in the midline, advance it further until resistance is felt and it locates in the back of the pharynx.
- Inflate the cuff with the appropriate amount of air. The tube should lift 1–2 cm out of the mouth as the cuff finds its correct position on inflation.
- Connect the tube to a bag-valve device with supplemental oxygen and confirm adequate ventilation by noting bilateral chest movement. Use a stethoscope to listen for air entry during ventilation.
- If placement of the LMA does not allow adequate ventilation within 30 seconds of commencement, it should be removed and the patient ventilated and oxygenated prior to further attempts.
- Insert a bite block, such as a roll of gauze or oropharyngeal airway, alongside the tube and tie the tube securely.

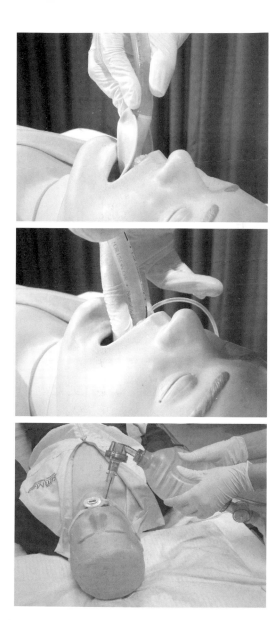

Fig. 7.5 Insertion of an LMA.

Combitube

At the time of writing, the Combitube is not widely used in the UK, in contrast to North America and many parts of Europe. However, its use may become more common as it offers similar appeal to the LMA in terms of training and skill requirements. For that reason it is mentioned only briefly (AHA & ILCOR 2000).

The Combitube is a rigid double-lumen tube that is inserted blindly into the patient's mouth and advanced towards the larynx. In the majority of cases the tube enters the patient's oesophagus but the design of the tube caters for the occasion when it may directly enter the trachea. The Combitube has a series of perforations and inflatable cuffs and due to the double lumen, the healthcare professional trained in its use would assess which port to ventilate by, depending on whether the device had lodged itself in the oesophagus or trachea. The Combitube and equipment necessary for its insertion are as shown in Figure 7.6.

VENTILATION

The patient who is not breathing or breathing inadequately will require assisted ventilation (Wenzel *et al.* 2001). This can be achieved by:

- mouth-to-mouth (nose) ventilation;
- mouth-to-mask ventilation;
- bag-valve device (attached to facemask, laryngeal mask airway, Combitube, endotracheal tube);
- automatic, mechanical ventilators.

Table 7.3 LMA cuff inflation volumes.

LMA size	Patient size	Cuff inflation
3	Small adult	Up to 20 ml
4	Medium adult	Up to 30 ml
5	Large adult	Up to 40 ml

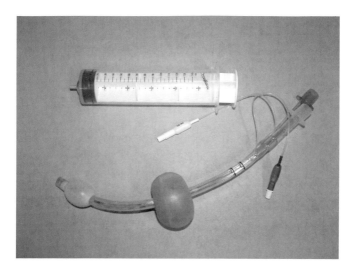

Fig. 7.6 The Combitube.

Mouth-to-mouth (nose) ventilation

Simple barrier devices such as faceshields are available to prevent direct mouth-to-mouth (nose) contact (Wenzel *et al.* 2001). These are usually plastic or silicone sheet-type devices that often have a one-way valve system. Some of them have a small tube that should be inserted into the patient's mouth whilst ensuring that it is not obstructed by the tongue. Mouth-to-faceshield breathing is continued in the same manner as mouth-to-mouth breathing (see Chapter 5).

Mouth-to-mask ventilation

The pocket mask is an excellent device that allows effective ventilation of a patient by less experienced personnel (Baskett *et al.* 1996). The mask provides protection to the rescuer through a one-way valve system. The pocket resuscitation mask is an anatomically shaped facemask with a cushioned under-edge. Most are marked to guide positioning of the mask on the patient's face. Some masks have an oxygen inlet, which allows supplemental oxygen to be given in addition to the rescuer's breaths. If no oxygen inlet is present, supplemental oxygen may still be administered by placing the oxygen tubing directly under the mask. There must be a good seal between the mask and the patient's face.

Technique
Ideally the patient should be in a supine position.

- Remove the mask from its container and form it into the correct shape by pushing the dome part forward (see Figure 7.7).
- Attach the one-way valve to the mouthpiece.
- Wear the gloves that are provided in the pocket mask container.
- Standing beside the patient or behind the patient's head, apply the mask to the patient's face. Use the bridge of the nose as a guide for correct placement.
- Apply firm pressure onto the cushioned part of the mask using your fingers and/or thumbs in a position that is comfortable and ensures a good seal between the mask and the patient's face.
- Perform head tilt/chin lift to open the airway.
- Blow gently through the one-way valve and look for chest movement. The chest should rise as with normal breathing. It is not necessary for the rescuer to deliver large breaths to effectively ventilate the patient's lungs.
- Allow the patient to exhale between each ventilation. Watch for the chest to fall before giving the next breath.
- Be aware that it may be difficult to get an adequate seal on the first attempt. In this situation reposition fingers and thumbs, adjust the mask and be sure the airway is opened correctly.
- An oral airway may be used to assist in maintaining the airway when using the pocket mask. However, attempted ventilation should not be delayed if one is not immediately available.
- Once oxygen is available, it should be attached to the oxygen inlet at a flow rate of 10 litres per minute. It is still necessary for the rescuer to blow into the mask to provide ventilation (see Figure 7.8).

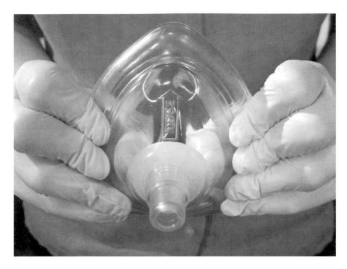

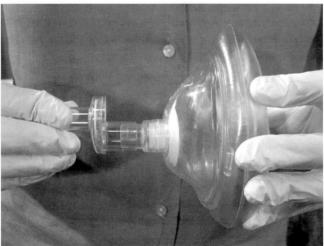

Fig. 7.7 Assembly of pocket mask.

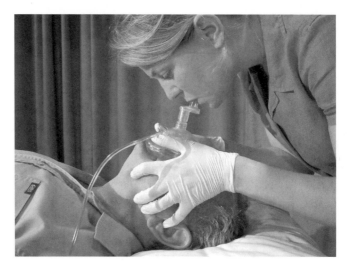

Fig. 7.8 Mouth-to-mask ventilation with additional oxygen attached.

Bag-valve device

Different sized facemasks
- The facial anatomy of casualties will always vary and so it is important to have a selection of suitable facemask sizes. The facemask will attach to the bag-valve system and a good seal will need to be achieved for effective ventilation.
- The facemasks should be made of clear material so that the operator may observe any blood or vomit coming from the patient's airway.

Technique
A two-person technique is recommended when using the bag-valve device with a facemask (Resuscitation Council UK 2000). One rescuer should hold the mask securely in place whilst maintaining a head tilt/chin lift position. The second rescuer should squeeze the bag gently to inflate the casualty's lungs (see Figure 7.9).

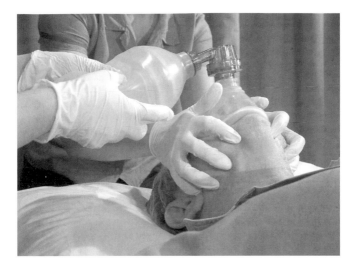

Fig. 7.9 Two-person bag-valve-mask ventilation.

The recommended tidal volumes for ventilations given with a bag-valve device with supplemental oxygen are 6–7 ml/kg (Resuscitation Council UK 2000). This tidal volume should provide normal chest movement in the casualty. Table 7.4 offers a guide for delivering supplementary oxygen.

Automatic mechanical ventilators

Automatic mechanical ventilators may be a useful adjunct during cardiopulmonary resuscitation, particularly in the pre-hospital setting where rescue times will be longer.

The ventilator is a small device that is often powered by the same oxygen cylinder which supplies the patient with oxygen. It works by providing a constant flow of gas to the patient during inspiration and has in-built pressure limitation controls. Considerable training is required and its use would therefore not be appropriate for an occasional user (Resuscitation Council UK 2000).

Table 7.4 Oxygen delivery guide.

Ventilatory device	Oxygen flow rate	Approximate oxygen concentration
Mouth-to-mouth (or nose)	Nil	16–17%
Mouth-to-mask	Nil	16–17%
Mouth-to-mask	10 l/min	40% or more
Bag-valve-mask (with no reservoir system attached)	Nil	21%
Bag-valve-mask (with reservoir system attached)	10–15 l/min	85%
Bag-valve-tube (LMA, ETT, Combitube) with reservoir system attached	10–15 l/min	Up to 100%

ADVANCED AIRWAY CONTROL AND VENTILATION: TRACHEAL INTUBATION

Intubation of the trachea with a cuffed tube is still considered to be the best possible means of maintaining a clear and secure airway in the cardiac arrest casualty (AHA & ILCOR 2000). However, whether or not this will result in an improved chance of survival for the casualty has not yet been proven through a prospective randomised trial. The current ALS algorithm (see Chapter 6) does not specify that intubation is necessary (Resuscitation Council UK 2000). Instead it stresses the importance of adequate ventilation and oxygenation.

Advantages of tracheal intubation

- Isolates the airway and prevents foreign material from entering the oropharynx.
- Provides a means of suctioning inhaled debris from the lower airway.
- Ventilation can generally be achieved without leaks, even if there is airway resistance.
- Prescribed tidal volumes can be delivered.
- It can be used as an alternative route to administer drugs if intravenous access has not been achieved.

Disadvantages of tracheal intubation

- Intubation requires extensive training and regular practice to maintain the skill.
- Numerous complications can arise as a result of tracheal intubation being attempted by unskilled operators, such as ventilation being withheld for unacceptable periods whilst intubation is repeatedly 'attempted'. Failure to oxygenate and ventilate results in death.
- It is important that any healthcare professional who may assist with intubation is fully conversant with the equipment necessary for this procedure (see Chapter 3).

REVIEW OF LEARNING

- ❏ Recognising airway and breathing problems promptly and responding with appropriate interventions will ensure hypoxic damage to vital organs is minimised.
- ❏ Airway obstruction may be partial or complete. The tongue is the most common form of airway obstruction in a patient with a decreased level of consciousness.
- ❏ The best way to recognise any degree of airway obstruction is to assess the patient by looking, listening and feeling.
- ❏ Often the basic airway opening manoeuvres of head tilt, chin lift and jaw thrust will be all that is required to relieve airway obstruction caused by the tongue.
- ❏ Oropharyngeal and nasopharyngeal airways are simple adjuncts that help to prevent backward displacement of the tongue in an unconscious patient.
- ❏ The LMA is an extremely reliable device that can be used during a resuscitation attempt for a patient who has become unconscious and stopped breathing.
- ❏ Assisted ventilation can be achieved by several methods including mouth-to-mouth or nose, mouth-to-mask, bag-valve device attached to facemask, LMA or endotracheal tube or automatic machanical ventilator.
- ❏ Where possible, oxygen should be administered with any ventilation attempts. Failure to do so may compromise chances of survival.
- ❏ The best way to ensure adequate ventilation in the patient is to assess by looking, listening and feeling.

Case study

Mrs Betty Booth is a 68-year-old lady who has been admitted to the ward for observation. She has taken an over-dose of sedative drugs. Considering her diagnosis, this patient may be at risk for airway and breathing compromise.

Make a list of potential causes of airway and breathing difficulties in such a patient. In addition, discuss how you would recognise any deterioration in Mrs Booth's condition.

- Central nervous system depression following the over-dose may result in loss of airway control
- Hypoxia
- Vomiting
- Regurgitation of gastric contents
- Loose dentures
- Saliva

The best way to recognise an airway or breathing problem is to:

- *look* for signs of a clear airway, level of responsiveness, skin colour and evidence of laboured breathing;
- *listen*, to determine whether the patient's breathing is noisy, silent or effortless and quiet;
- *feel* for signs of exhaled air.

Following your assessment of Mrs Booth, you find that she is now difficult to arouse. She is pale and clammy with shallow breathing at a rate of approximately six breaths per minute. You can hear gurgling coming from her airway. **How would you respond?**

- Open the airway using head tilt and chin lift.
- Use suction to clear the mouth.
- Administer high-flow oxygen via a non-rebreathe oxygen mask.
- Consider inserting an oropharyngeal or nasopharyngeal airway.
- Consider calling the medical emergency team.

Continued

Whilst you are managing the situation you recognise that Mrs Booth has become completely unresponsive and has stopped breathing. A pulse check reveals bradycardia at 45 beats per minute. **How will you respond to this further deterioration?**

Call for appropriate help. If an LMA is immediately available and you are competent in its use then insert it without pre-oxygenation. If the LMA is not an option then begin to ventilate the patient using a mouth-to-mask or bag-valve-mask technique with supplemental oxygen attached. Aim to provide ventilations at a normal respiratory rate (approx 12 breaths per minute). Monitor the effectiveness of ventilations using the look, listen and feel approach. Consider further monitoring, i.e. pulse oximetry and electrocardiogram, to recognise any further deterioration in the circulatory system. Whilst the patient is in respiratory arrest, continue to check the pulse every minute.

CONCLUSION

This chapter has considered the management of airway and breathing in the compromised casualty. The guidelines for delivery are designed to aid recall and support effective resuscitation and all healthcare professionals should be familiar with the most up-to-date guidelines, by regularly accessing the *Resuscitation* journal and Resuscitation Council UK and European Resuscitation Council websites (www.resus.org.uk and www.erc.edu).

REFERENCES

American Heart Association and International Liaison Committee on Resuscitation (2000) Part 6. Adjuncts for oxygenation, ventilation, and airway control. *Circulation* **102** (suppl I), 95–104.

Baskett, P.J.F., Bossaert, L., Chamberlain, D. *et al.* (1996) Guidelines for the basic management of the airway and ventilation during resuscitation. A statement by the airway and ventilation management working group of the European Resuscitation Council. *Resuscitation* **31**, 187–200.

Resuscitation Council UK (2000) *Advanced Life Support Course Provider Manual*, 4th edn. Resuscitation Council UK, London.

Stone, B.J., Chantler, P.J. & Baskett, P.J.F. (1998) The incidence of regurgitation during cardiopulmonary resuscitation: a comparison between the bag valve mask and laryngeal mask airway. *Resuscitation* **3**, 3–7.

Wenzel, V., Idris, A.H., Dorges, V. *et al.* (2001) The respiratory system during resuscitation: a review of the history, risk of infection during assisted ventilation, respiratory mechanics, and ventilation strategies for patients with an unprotected airway. *Resuscitation* **49**, 123–34.

Monitoring and Assessing Cardiac Rhythms

8

INTRODUCTION

Increasingly healthcare staff are expected to manage the care of patients who may be at risk of developing life-threatening arrhythmias. To recognise and respond to life-threatening arrhythmias demands skill and knowledge as well as understanding of the effects that non-cardiac disorders have on the electrocardiograph (ECG) (Meek & Morris 2002a).

Interpreting normal and abnormal cardiac rhythms requires detailed appreciation of the conducting system. In becoming familiar with the underlying concepts of electro-cardiography and cardiac monitoring techniques, healthcare professionals can start to accurately differentiate rhythm disturbances that may suggest compromised cardiovascular function, myocardial irritability or instability which may precipitate a cardiac arrest.

AIMS

This chapter introduces the concepts associated with cardiac monitoring and discusses each of the main shockable, non-shockable and peri-arrest rhythms.

LEARNING OUTCOMES

By the end of this chapter the reader should be able to:

❏ describe the *electrical conduction system of the heart*;
❏ discuss the *principles of cardiac monitoring*;
❏ explain the *main components of sinus rhythm*;
❏ describe the *physiological characteristics of shockable rhythms* and treatments;
❏ describe the *physiological characteristics of non-shockable rhythms and peri-arrest rhythms* and respective treatments.

ELECTRICAL CONDUCTION PATHWAYS OF THE HEART

Understanding the electrical activity of the heart is key to developing an appreciation of changes in the ECG.

Conducting system

- Electrical activity begins with pacemaker cells of the sino-atrial (SA) node. Here, cells are able to generate a spontaneous impulse without nervous innervation and normally determine the heart rate.
- Once the SA node depolarises, waves of electrical activity travel across the right and left atria, causing these chambers to contract.
- The impulses then reach the atrioventricular (AV) node, where there is a brief period of delayed conduction.
- Impulses are then propagated downwards in a co-ordinated fashion, initially along the atrioventricular bundle of His.
- The bundle consists of specialised conducting tissue that divides into the right and left bundle branches.
- The bundle of His and bundle branches are central to the propagation of impulses, which eventually terminate in fine branches or Purkinje fibres.
- The Purkinje fibres are embedded in ventricular myocardium and these will transmit impulses to the ventricular muscle mass, resulting in contraction. Ventricles comprise a large muscle mass and are able to generate spontaneous impulses but at a slower rate than pacemaker cells, namely at a rate of 20–40 beats per minute (bpm) (Meek & Morris 2000a).

The spread of impulses from cell to cell and across the entire heart is known as 'depolarisation', whereas the stage of 're-polarisation' relates to myocardial recovery. In practice, the 'electrical' cycle of the heart can be fully assessed by a 12-lead ECG from the patient. Specifically, an ECG machine measures and records, on graph-like paper, voltage variations (of the atria and ventricles) plotted against time. These waves of electrical activity have three distinctive features.

Duration

The time element that is measured along the horizontal axis and in fractions of a second.

- 1 small square equals 0.04 sec or 1 mm in width.
- 1 large square equals 0.2 sec or 5 mm in width.
- 300 large squares represent one minute.

Amplitude
A voltage component that is measured along the vertical axis in millivolts.

- 1 small square equals 0.1 mv or 1 mm.
- 1 large square equals 0.5 mv or 5 mm.

Composition
This relates to specific arrangements in the waves in terms of shape and appearance.

PRINCIPLES OF CARDIAC MONITORING
The ECG displayed on the monitor screen must be clear and well defined to avoid misdiagnosis or inappropriate treatment. A cardiac trace can be obtained through three or five colour-coded ECG leads that are attached to electrodes placed on the anterior surface of a patient's chest. Signals emitted from the heart are sensed from the skin surface by the electrodes and are subsequently transmitted, by means of a cable, to the cardiac monitor, which in turn magnifies them into recognisable waves. The displayed image reflects one view and while single-lead monitoring remains widely used, it has limited value in the diagnosis of other clinical conditions. However, modern monitors are multipurpose and permit a range of functions including continuous transmission of leads I, II, III (see Figure 8.1), as well as displaying non-invasive blood pressure and oxygen saturation readings. It is also possible to configure the technology to display 12-lead ECG and ST segment monitoring options.

Defibrillator paddles and gel pads can also be used to monitor a cardiac rhythm, particularly when the cardiac arrest is not witnessed. It is the quickest way to assess whether the casualty is in a shockable rhythm. Automated external defibrillators require application of large adhesive multipurpose electrodes to the casualty's chest, which allow for monitoring of cardiac rhythm and defibrillation.

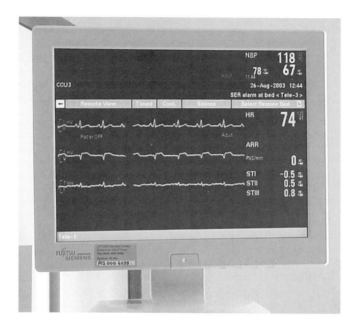

Fig. 8.1 Monitor displays three leads and ST segment monitoring.

Lead placement

The Resuscitation Council UK (2000) recommends that for the purposes of monitoring, lead II should be selected as it provides the clearest view of the P wave and the QRS complex. A lead II trace is obtained by placing the red (positive) electrode on the right shoulder, the yellow (negative) electrode on the left shoulder and the black or green (neutral) electrode below the left border of the ribcage.

To ensure a high-quality ECG trace, consider the following principles.

- Maintain good skin contact (remove chest hair as it may interfere with adhesion of electrodes to skin).
- Keep skin surface dry (rub the sites selected for placement of electrodes with dry gauze).

- Apply even pressure only on adhesive area to ensure a good seal.
- Avoid placing electrodes where defibrillation gel pads might be positioned in the event of a cardiac arrest.
- Avoid interference from patient movement, electrical equipment and during CPR by attaching the ECG electrodes over bone rather than muscle.
- Apply large adhesive multipurpose electrodes as recommended.
- Check ECG or replace electrodes if trace is poor or interrupted.
- Set alarms for upper and lower limits of heart rate in line with local practice.
- Record the patient's details, symptoms, date and time alongside the trace or ECG recording.

Problems encountered during cardiac monitoring

There are many factors that may affect the quality of the ECG trace appearing on the cardiac monitor so knowing how to minimise or prevent such problems is vital (Jevon 2003). Good practice involves always assessing the patient first before the equipment.

Straight/flat-line
- Assess for evidence of cable damage.
- Check that all equipment is connected correctly.
- Ensure the gain has been set appropriately.
- Make sure lead II has been selected.
- Check electrodes are in date and intact.
- Check other leads.

Quality of the ECG trace is inadequate
- Review connections and cable.
- Assess that electrodes have been correctly placed.
- Check that the electrodes have not become displaced.
- Electrodes are in date and intact.
- Replace electrodes.

Wandering baseline and artefacts
- Voluntary artefact – can be caused by patient movement such as respiration. Consider moving electrodes.
- Involuntary artefact – includes interference caused by shivering or nervousness. Keep patient warm and provide emotional support.
- Electrical interference – this is due to electrical equipment such as infusion pumps and syringe drivers. Ensure minimal contact with cardiac leads.
- Loose electrode – a wandering baseline pattern suggests signal interruption due to a loose electrode, poor contact or incorrectly placed electrode.
- Complexes are too small – these may be due to clinical factors such as a cardiac tamponade or pericardial effusion. Select a different lead, increase amplitude or substitute electrodes.
- False heart rate on display – occasionally the ECG complexes appear as very small on the cardiac monitor, giving the impression of a reduced heart rate. At other times the T wave may be counted for an R wave, thus doubling the heart rate. Reposition electrodes or select another lead to correct this problem (Jevon 2003).

COMPONENTS OF SINUS RHYTHM

Heart rate
Heart rate can be influenced by sympathetic and parasympathetic activity. Other factors that influence the heart rate include stimulants (nicotine, caffeine), drugs (beta-blockers) and conditions such as thyrotoxicosis and hypoxia. In health, the heart's resting rhythm is regular although the rate varies between 60 and 99 beats per minute (Meek & Morris 2002a).

Rhythm
Sinus rhythm is the term given to a rhythm that is regular, originates in the sinoatrial node, with a heart rate of 60–99 beats per minute. Sinus bradycardia is similar but the rate is below 60 whereas with sinus tachycardia, the rate is between 100 and 130 bpm.

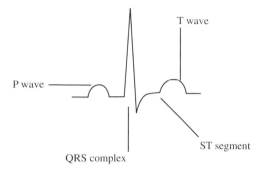

Fig. 8.2 The PQRST waves of a sinus rhythm complex.

Characteristic features of sinus rhythm

- The P wave – is produced by atrial depolarisation. As the atria possess little muscle, the P wave is small. The P wave is best seen in lead II and VI where it is normally a positive deflection. Its shape is rounded and smooth and is less than 0.12 sec in duration (see Figure 8.2).
- The PR interval – represents the time it takes for the impulse to travel from the SA node to the AV node and the bundle of His and cause ventricular contraction, normally 0.12–0.20 sec (see Table 8.1).
- The QRS complex – represents the spread of impulses by the ventricles. The R wave is the first upward deflection after the P wave. The height of the R wave is variable in different leads but the normal QRS width should be less than 0.12 sec or three little squares.
- The ST segment – usually runs fairly flat along the isoelectric line. It signifies the end of ventricular depolarisation and the start of electrical recovery. A rise of 1 mm in either standard or limb leads or a 2 mm rise in the precordial leads is associated with ischaemia or infarction.
- The T wave – confirms that repolarisation has taken place. The T wave should be upright in I, II, AVF, V3–V6, inverted in AVR as well as leads III and VI and variable in the remaining leads. The shape of the T wave is usually smooth and rounded.

Table 8.1 Normal PQRST intervals (Jevon 2003, Meek & Morris 2002b).

Interval	Duration	Measurement	Abnormality
PR interval	0.12–0.20 sec	From the start of the P wave to the first deflection of QRS	If prolonged, consider delayed or abnormal conduction
QRS interval	0.08–0.12 sec	Begins at the Q wave and ends with the S wave deflection	If QRS is >0.12 sec consider abnormalities in conduction such as bundle branch block or ventricular arrhythmia. A QRS complex that is <0.12 sec will be narrow in shape and originate above the ventricles
QT interval	0.35–0.45 sec	From the beginning of QRS until the end of the T wave	Prolonged QT interval is due to hypothermia, drugs and electrolyte disorders such as calcium; may need to be adjusted for age and gender

SHOCKABLE RHYTHMS

Ventricular tachycardia

Ventricular tachycardia (VT) is confirmed by five or more ventricular ectopics in succession and it is usually accompanied by a sudden onset of signs and symptoms. If this rhythm occurs post myocardial infarction it can degenerate into ventricular fibrillation (VF). Ventricular tachycardia can be triggered by an irritable site within the ventricles; conduction takes place across ventricular cells, rather than along the normal specialised conducting pathway, resulting in the broad shape of the complexes. A broad complex suggests that it originates in the ventricles, particularly if the QRS complex exceeds 0.16 sec.

Causes
- Ischaemic heart disease (IHD) and myocardial infarction
- Hypertrophic obstructive cardiomyopathy
- Electrolyte disturbances
- Drug toxicity or use of recreational drugs such as cocaine
- Mechanical stimulation from pacing wire or invasive line

Characteristic features of the ECG (Figure 8.3)
- P wave may be present in some leads and not in others.
- QRS rate between 150 and 300/min.
- QRS rhythm may be regular or almost regular, unless fusion beats present.
- QRS broad and wide (>0.12 sec or longer).
- Presence of atrioventricular dissociation (Edhouse & Morris 2002a).
- There is concordance across the chest leads, meaning that all QRS complexes are either positively or negatively orientated.

Clinical features
Most patients will present with symptoms associated with coronary artery disease or haemodynamic instability due to poor tissue perfusion. Symptoms may include palpitations, chest pain, profuse sweating and anxiety. The patient may lose consciousness due to a reduced cardiac output.

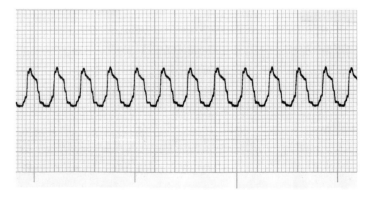

Fig. 8.3 Ventricular tachycardia.

Response
- If the patient is tolerating the rhythm, seek expert assistance and attempt emergency cardioversion if response to drugs is unsuccessful (European Resuscitation Council (ERC) 2001).
- If no signs of life, follow the advanced life support algorithm for VF and pulseless VT (see Chapter 6).

Other facts
- VT can be self-terminating or 'non-sustained' when it returns to a normal rhythm within 30 seconds.
- In regular or monomorphic VT, the most common form of this arrhythmia, the appearance between beats is the same.
- In irregular or polymorphic VT (torsade de pointes tachycardia), there is wide beat-to-beat variation in the QRS morphology rotating every 5–20 beats along the baseline (Spearritt 2003). Torsade de pointes represents an uncommon variant form of VT which may deteriorate into VF. It may occur after a myocardial infarction or be associated with prolonged repolarisation known as QT syndromes. IHD, hypomagnesaemia, antiarrhythmics, antibacterials and bradycardia due to sick sinus syndrome precipitate torsade des pointes (Edhouse & Morris 2002b). Treatment involves alleviating any predisposing cause, improving electrolyte imbalance and overdrive pacing (Bennett 2002, Resuscitation Council UK 2000).

Ventricular fibrillation
Ventricular fibrillation is often referred to as chaotic and uncoordinated electrical activity; it is triggered by thousands of ventricular foci discharging at different and rapid rates (shown in Figure 8.4). The lack of a strong ventricular contraction causes circulatory collapse and loss of consciousness.

Causes
- Myocardial ischaemia (may occur after myocardial infarction or be associated with a prolonged QT interval)
- Electrolyte disorders such as potassium
- Cardiomyopathy
- Accidental electrical shock
- Digoxin toxicity
- Hypothermia

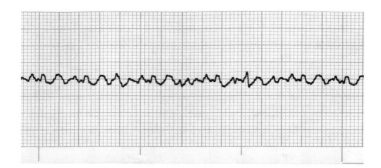

Fig. 8.4 Ventricular fibrillation.

Clinical features
The patient will experience a loss of consciousness, become pulseless and cease breathing.

Characteristic features of the ECG
- P wave and PR interval are unrecognisable.
- QRS rate and rhythm are not definable.
- QRS complex is not discernible.
- There is a wavy line composed of different waves whose amplitude and appearance are variable.
- In the early stages of VF the appearance is coarse but after some minutes it becomes progressively smaller or 'fine VF'. Fine VF can resemble asystole; to distinguish this, increase the gain on the monitor or review the rhythm in a different lead.

Response
Follow the algorithm for VF and aim to defibrillate the casualty within three minutes of collapsing once cardiac arrest has been confirmed.

NON-SHOCKABLE RHYTHMS
Asystole and pulseless electrical activity (PEA) present as clinical emergencies as they are both life-threatening rhythms. The

outcome for these non-shockable rhythms is poor unless the underlying factors can be identified and treated promptly and effectively.

Asystole

Asystole is characterised by complete absence of electrical activity within the heart (see Figure 8.5). According to Gwinnutt *et al.* (2000), asystole is present in 25% of in-hospital cardiac arrests.

Causes
- Extensive coronary artery ischaemia
- Myocardial infarction
- Hypoxia
- Electrolyte imbalance
- Drug toxicity
- Prolonged episode of VF

Clinical features
The patient will suffer a cardiac arrest, lose consciousness, become pulseless and cease breathing.

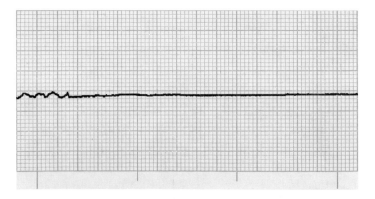

Fig. 8.5 Asystole.

Characteristic features of the ECG
- No ECG waveform is recognisable so there is no sign of a rate or a rhythm.
- If only the P waves are present, the rhythm is described as ventricular standstill.
- A flat baseline or trace may appear (this must be differentiated from fine VF). Asystole must be established by reviewing the leads and checking they are attached to the patient, increasing the gain and comparing the rhythm through two different leads (Jevon 2003).
- Spurious asystole (after multiple defibrillations) must be excluded if reading through paddles; instead ECG leads should be used for monitoring (Resuscitation Council UK 2000).

Response
- Confirm that patient is in asystole.
- Commence basic life support (BLS) for three minutes (15:2) if patient is arrested.
- Follow right-sided path of ALS algorithm (ERC 2001; also see Chapter 6).

Pulseless electrical activity (PEA)
In PEA the clinical features of a cardiac arrest are present but there are also regular or near regular complexes displayed on the screen although the cardiac output is absent. Data from Gwinnutt *et al.* (2000) suggest that PEA features in approximately 35% of all in-hospital arrests. There are two forms of PEA, primary and secondary (Jevon 2003).

- Primary PEA – brought on by myocardial fibres not contracting effectively, resulting in the loss of cardiac output. Normally associated with large MI, drugs, calcium channel blockers, poisoning and electrolyte disturbances including hyperkalaemia and hypocalcaemia.
- Secondary PEA – the result of a mechanical problem that impedes ventricular filling or ejection. The causes include ventricular wall rupture, hypovolaemia, tension pneumothorax, pulmonary embolism and cardiac tamponade.

Clinical features
- Absence of a carotid pulse.
- Physical signs of a cardiac arrest.

Characteristic features of the ECG
Evidence of electrical activity in the form of a regular or irregular rhythm on the cardiac monitor, which is associated with signs of cardiac arrest and the absence of a cardiac output. The patient may present with a rhythm such as atrial fibrillation.

Response
- Confirm patient has arrested; if no signs of life, institute BLS immediately.
- Begin aggressive searching for the cause of the arrest.
- Treatment involves following the right side path of the ALS algorithm (ERC 2001; see Chapter 6).
- Consider and correct reversible causes (see Chapter 11).

PERI-ARREST ARRHYTHMIAS

Peri-arrest rhythms are those that may present as emergency situations. Many of these adverse arrhythmias occur following a myocardial infarction, resuscitation or other factors. In such instances, if standard measures to manage or prevent arrhythmias are ineffective, expert help should be sought promptly (ERC 2001).

Adverse arrhythmias can manifest with the following signs and symptoms.

- Evidence of a low cardiac output – for example, hypotension, cool peripheries, clamminess, pallor, confusion.
- Excessive tachycardias – a narrow or broad complex tachycardia can significantly decrease diastolic time, resulting in impaired coronary blood flow and myocardial ischaemia.
- Excessive bradycardias – usually defined as a rate less than 40 bpm, although some patients may become symptomatic at higher rates.
- Cardiac failure – includes the triad of pulmonary oedema, a raised jugular venous pressure and hepatic engorgement (ERC 2001).

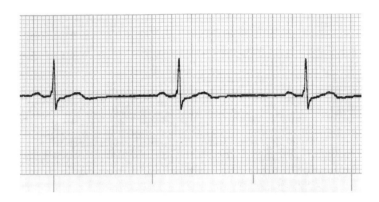

Fig. 8.6 Bradycardia.

The major peri-arrest rhythms include:

- bradycardia
- atrial fibrillation
- other narrow complex tachycardia
- broad complex tachycardia.

Bradycardia

In general terms a heart rate of less than 60 beats per minute is an arbitrary figure used to describe a bradycardic rhythm, although there are many healthy individuals, such as athletes, who are clinically well despite having a slow heart rate (Da Costa *et al.* 2002). A profound bradycardia (see Figure 8.6) may occur due to a cardiac or non-cardiac disorder and is of importance if the following changes occur:

- a systolic blood pressure <90 mmHg;
- a pulse rate of <40 beats per minute;
- ventricular arrhythmias requiring suppression;
- heart failure.

Causes
- Hypothermia.
- Drugs (beta-blockers, some calcium channel blockers, digoxin).

- Hypothyroidism.
- Sick sinus syndrome.
- Electrolyte disorders.
- Patients with inferior myocardial infarctions are prone to suffer from a bradycardic episode, due to the involvement of the right coronary artery.

If there are adverse signs, intravenous atropine 500 µg should be administered. If the response is positive or if there are no adverse signs present, then assess for risk of asystole. Those at risk include people with:

- recent history of asystole;
- Mobitz type II atrioventricular block;
- ventricular pause greater than three seconds;
- complete heart block with a wide QRS (as seen in Figure 8.7).

Characteristic features of the ECG
These will depend on the underlying rhythm.

- Slow heart rates.
- P waves may appear regularly or intermittently.
- Variable regular or irregular ventricular rates.

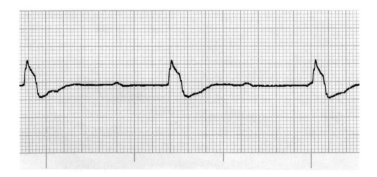

Fig. 8.7 Complete heart block.

Response
- Intravenous atropine 500 µg repeated up to a maximum of 3 mg.
- If pacing is unavailable, titrated low-dose epinephrine infusion in the range 2–10 µg/min is recommended instead.
- Transvenous (external) pacing, particularly if the risk of asystole is high (ERC 2001, Resuscitation Council UK 2000).

Atrial fibrillation

Atrial fibrillation (AF) is one of the most common dysrhythmias with a prevalence of 1–1.5%, a figure that increases with advancing age. AF is characterised by erratic, disorganised and chaotic atrial activity that is associated with an irregular ventricular response which helps maintain cardiac output. The rhythm is triggered by multiple atrial ectopic foci stimulated at a frequency of 350–600 beats per minute outside the SA node region (Goodacre & Irons 2002). However, conduction down the His–Purkinje system is random and intermittent, resulting in an irregular ventricular response noted in the ECG. Since atrial contractions are weak, the potential for pooling and thrombus formation is strong, particularly in those who have experienced AF for more than 24 hours (Hand 2002).

The ERC (2001) treatment guidelines on peri-arrest arrhythmias classify AF according to whether it is high, intermediate (see Figure 8.8) or low risk. This division depends on the rate of AF and the presenting signs and symptoms.

Table 8.2 Atrial fibrillation risk.

Intermediate risk	High risk
• Heart rate 100–150	• Heart rate greater than 150 bpm
• Dyspnoea	• Ongoing chest pain
• Poor tissue perfusion	• Critical tissue perfusion

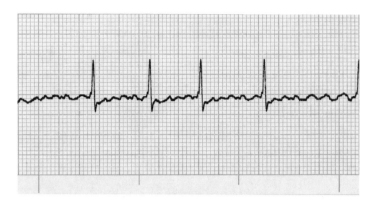

Fig. 8.8 Atrial fibrillation.

Causes

- Digoxin toxicity
- Post valve surgery
- Hypertension
- Increased sympathetic activity
- IHD

- Chronic pulmonary disease
- Acute or chronic alcohol misuse
- Thyrotoxicosis
- Cardiomyopathies

- Rheumatic valve disease

Clinical presentation
The patient may experience palpitations, shortness of breath, syncope or chest pain and a reduced cardiac output.

Characteristic features of the ECG
- P waves are absent; instead oscillating f (fibrillation) wavelets can be seen (Figure 8.8).
- PR interval not measurable.
- Atrial rate may be very rapid and difficult to determine.
- No identifiable relationship between the P waves and QRS complexes.
- QRS rate may be slow or fast and the rhythm will be irregular.
- QRS width is within normal parameters (Goodacre & Irons 2002).

Response

Treatment options for those classified as intermediate risk take into account evidence of haemodynamic status, whether the onset of AF occurred within 24 hours and the presence of structural heart disease (ERC 2001). A heparin infusion followed by emergency electrical cardioversion (see Chapter 9) should be considered for high-risk patients. If cardioversion is unsuccessful or AF recurs, intravenous amiodarone 300 mg should be administered over one hour before attempting cardioversion again (Resuscitation Council UK 2000). Management also involves addressing the reversible causes immediately, aiming to:

- control the rate by slowing ventricular response;
- control rhythm by conversion to sinus rhythm;
- restore haemodynamic functioning and circulation;
- maintain sinus rhythm and prevent further episodes.

The time of onset and haemodynamic stability of the patient are variables which will affect treatment decisions (ERC 2001).

Narrow complex tachycardias

Narrow complex tachycardias, for example, supraventricular tachycardia (SVT, as shown in Figure 8.9), are triggered by an ectopic focus situated above the ventricles, which results in impulses being conducted rapidly along the specialised cells in the intraventricular septum. Because SVT originates above the AV node, the QRS complex will be narrow (<0.12 sec). In extreme cases narrow complex tachycardias can also have a profound effect on cardiac output, resulting in the loss of cardiac output and impaired consciousness. Edhouse & Morris (2002b) also suggest that SVT is more likely to occur in those under 35 years of age.

Causes
- Rheumatic heart disease
- Cardiomyopathy
- Ischaemic heart disease
- Pericarditis
- Hypertension
- Thyrotoxicosis
- Pulmonary embolism

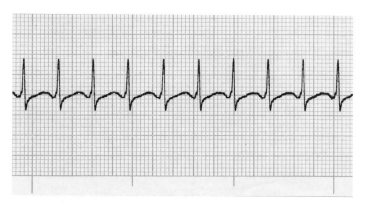

Fig. 8.9 A narrow complex tachycardia.

Clinical presentation
- Patients may be clammy and hypotensive and experience chest pain and palpitations.
- Rhythm may be precipitated by stress or alcohol.
- The rhythm may have an abrupt onset and termination.

Characteristic features of the ECG
Narrow complex tachycardia, presumed to be SVT.

- P waves are not always detectable.
- PR interval is not measurable.
- The relationship between P waves and QRS complex is not discernible.
- There is a QRS rate of 150–250 beats per minute.
- QRS rate tends to be regular.
- QRS complex tends to be narrow (<0.12 sec), unlike VT.
- V leads are discordant (some are positive and others negative) on examination of the 12-lead ECG.

Response
This is largely going to depend on the presenting rhythm and symptoms (ERC 2001).

- Administer oxygen and establish venous access.
- If the rhythm is indicative of AF, then see page 143.
- If the patient is pulseless, follow the left side of the algorithm.
- Vagal manoeuvres such as carotid sinus massage or Valsalva manoeuvre may terminate the narrow complex tachycardias and must only be attempted in the absence of contra-indications.
- In carotid sinus massage, the pulse has to be located and then massaged. If there is evidence of a carotid bruit this technique should be avoided due to possible complications; inexperienced personnel should not perform carotid sinus massage. Bradycardia is another side-effect of this technique.
- The Valsalva manoeuvre involves asking the patient to cough or to try to blow into a 20 ml syringe, inducing a strain effect which forces expiration against a closed glottis.
- If vagal stimulants fail, intravenous adenosine 6 mg may be administered rapidly in a bolus and flushed with saline. The effect of adenosine is to inhibit or slow conduction of impulses across the AV node. The patient should be warned that they might feel unpleasant sensations in the chest.
- Should the patient be symptomatic and unresponsive to vagal manoeuvres or adenosine and adverse signs and symptoms persist, synchronised cardioversion is recommended. In the presence of adverse signs, the patient must be sedated and synchronised cardioversion with 100 J, 200 J or 360 J should be delivered.

Broad complex tachycardias (presumed to be sustained VT)

These are normally considered to be of ventricular origin and treatment options include the following:

- If no pulse is present, follow VF/VT cardiac arrest algorithm.

- If pulse is present but the patient exhibits adverse clinical signs (chest pain, systolic BP <90 mmHg, heart failure or rate of >150 bpm), undertake synchronised cardioversion followed by intravenous amiodarone.
- If the patient is stable and able to tolerate the rhythm, anti-arrhythmic therapy with amiodarone through a central line should be started. Where this is unsuccessful, synchronised cardioversion may be necessary. Any electrolyte abnormalities should be corrected (Resuscitation Council UK 2000).

REVIEW OF LEARNING

❏ To be able to *recognise* and *respond* to potential and actual life-threatening arrhythmias, an understanding of the basic conduction system and the characteristics of sinus rhythm is essential.

❏ Prior to attaching the leads to the monitor, check that all equipment is in good working order and within date of expiry.

❏ Cardiac monitors, defibrillator paddles and AED adhesive electrodes can be used to assess the underlying rhythm.

❏ In general, the main rhythms that require emergency defibrillation are ventricular fibrillation and pulseless ventricular tachycardia.

❏ If the patient presents in asystole, it is important to check that all the leads are connected, the gain is increased to eliminate the possibility of fine VF and the rhythm is inspected in two other leads.

❏ Healthcare professionals must be suspicious of the patient who presents without a pulse but whose ECG reveals a regular and normal complex.

❏ Peri-arrest arrhythmias pose a risk to the patient. Knowledge of these rhythms, their prophylactic and emergency treatments will enhance the effectiveness of the healthcare professional.

❏ The ALS algorithm for the management of the adult in cardiac arrest provides guidance on treatment actions.

Case study

Mrs Wilson is a 67-year-old woman who arrives at your ward with a history of chest pain and episodes of feeling faint. After some formalities, you explain that you need to attach her to the monitor to obtain a continuous display of her heart rhythm. Mrs Wilson consents to the procedure and you draw the curtains.

How do you make certain that the ECG display on the monitor screen is of high quality?

Prior to starting, inspect the leads and the cable connected to the monitor, check for signs of damage and if soiled, clean before use. Check electrodes to make sure that they are in date and intact, then attach according to local practice. Ensure a good contact with the patient's skin. To avoid interference, make certain that the electrodes are placed over bone and to obtain good contact, make sure the skin is dry.

Place the ECG electrodes away from areas that could be used for defibrillation. If there is a poor signal replace the electrodes and check all connections as well as the lead for signs of damage. If the patient becomes clammy, change the electrodes more frequently. Should the complexes appear too small, check the patient, select another lead and increase the amplitude or replace electrodes. Finally, set the alarms and explain to the patient their significance and factors which may inadvertently set them off.

You note that Mrs Wilson's rhythm appears regular and the digital display indicates that her rate is 90 bpm. Discuss the features of: P, QRS, ST and T waves. For a complete answer, review the appropriate section of the chapter.

Whilst you are taking the history, Mrs Wilson complains of increasing chest pain. You reassure her and administer oxygen via mask. Whilst doing this you are aware that the non-invasive blood pressure has fallen to 90/60 mmHg, she has a tachycardia of more than 150 bpm and has become clammy.

Discuss the symptoms and ECG characteristics of ventricular tachycardia

In ventricular tachycardia the patient may or may not be responsive. In addition, the ECG will reveal key changes which can be found earlier in this chapter.

CONCLUSION

The ECG is a diagnostic tool used to assess cardiac rhythms continuously and provide an indication of changes within the heart's function. To be of value, healthcare staff must ensure that they are familiar with the techniques for ensuring that a high-quality ECG trace is displayed on the screen and know how to minimise artefacts and sources of interference. Being able to recognise shockable, non-shockable and peri-arrest rhythms and how to respond to these distinct forms of cardiac arrest also requires practice supported by undertaking additional educational input.

REFERENCES

Bennett, D.H. (2002) *Cardiac Arrhythmias: Practical Notes on Interpretation and Treatment*, 6th edn. Edward Arnold, London.

Da Costa, D., Brady, W.J. & Edhouse, J. (2002) ABC of clinical electrocardiography: bradycardias and atrioventricular conduction block. *British Medical Journal* **324**, 535–8.

Edhouse, J. & Morris, F. (2002a) ABC of clinical electrocardiography: broad complex tachycardia – part I. *British Medical Journal* **324**, 719–22.

Edhouse, J. & Morris, F. (2002b) ABC of clinical electrocardiography: broad complex tachycardia – part II. *British Medical Journal* **324**, 776–9.

European Resuscitation Council Guidelines for Adult Advanced Life Support (2001) A statement from the advanced life support working group and approved by the Executive Committee of the European Resuscitation Council. *Resuscitation* **48**, 211–21.

Goodacre, S. & Irons, R. (2002) ABC of clinical electrocardiography: atrial arrhythmias. *British Medical Journal* **324**, 594–7.

Gwinnutt, C., Coulumbo, M. & Harris, R. (2000) Outcome after cardiac arrest in adults in UK hospitals: effect of the 1997 guidelines. *Resuscitation* **47**, 125–35.

Hand, H. (2002) Common cardiac arrhythmias. *Nursing Standard* **16** (28), 43–52.

Jevon, P. (2003) *ECGs for Nurses*. Blackwell Publishing, Oxford.

Meek, S. & Morris, F. (2002a) Introduction I – leads, rate, rhythm and cardiac axis. *British Medical Journal* **324**, 415–18.

Meek, S. & Morris, F. (2002b) Introduction II – basic terminology. *British Medical Journal* **324**, 470–3.

Resuscitation Council UK (2000) *Advanced Life Support Provider Manual*, 4th edn. Resuscitation Council UK, London.

Spearritt, D. (2003) Torsade de pointes following cardioversion: case history and literature review. *Australian Critical Care* **16** (4), 144–9.

Defibrillation Theory and Practice

9

INTRODUCTION

Survival outcomes after a cardiac arrest depend on recognising the victim and responding with early defibrillation. Defibrillation remains the only clinically effective intervention for ventricular fibrillation (VF) and pulseless ventricular tachycardia (VT). Traditionally the skill of defibrillation has been confined to those working in critical care areas but advances in technology now make it possible for other healthcare professionals to learn how to defibrillate safely and effectively. Indeed, the introduction of smaller, lighter and easier to operate automated external defibrillators (AED) and advisory defibrillators that are highly sensitive and reliable has facilitated life-saving treatment to be rapidly available and provided by a range of hospital personnel.

In response to the role of early defibrillation in reducing mortality rates from VT/VF, the American Heart Association in collaboration with the International Liaison Committee on Resuscitation (AHA & ILCOR 2000) has issued guidelines for the use of AEDs as part of basic life support (BLS). The guidelines have been informed by the past three decades of research which have demonstrated an increase in survival rates from cardiac arrests following the early use of the AED by a number of health providers, first responders and lay people (Moule & Albarran 2002). Confidence in the ability of lay people and other rescuers to operate AEDs following minimal training resulted in recommendations by the European Resuscitation Council (Bossaert *et al.* 1998) and the Resuscitation Council UK (2000b) that all hospital and paramedic staff who may need to respond or may be witness to a cardiopulmonary emergency must be competent in BLS and be authorised to perform defibrillation using an AED.

AIMS
This chapter introduces the concepts of defibrillation and synchronised cardioversion and provides standardised guidance on how to operate a defibrillator safely and effectively.

LEARNING OUTCOMES
By the end of the chapter the reader should be able to:

❏ discuss the *basic principles and purpose of early defibrillation*;
❏ discuss the *factors that impact on successful defibrillation*;
❏ describe the key components in *operating a manual defibrillator*;
❏ describe the features and stages of *using automated external defibrillators* (AEDs);
❏ explain the principles and procedures associated with *synchronised cardioversion*;
❏ demonstrate knowledge of the *broad safety issues* when operating a defibrillator;
❏ describe the role and functions of *implantable cardiac defibrillators*.

PRINCIPLES AND PURPOSE OF EARLY DEFIBRILLATION
According to Gwinnutt *et al.* (2000), ventricular fibrillation and pulseless ventricular tachycardia are the initial presenting rhythm disturbances in about 30% of in-hospital cardiac arrests and in around 85% out-of-hospital arrests (Holmberg *et al.* 2000).

Patients with myocardial ischaemia or an infarction are most likely to experience an episode of VF or VT, which may be exacerbated by stress and cardiac pain. The release of circulating catecholamines, part of a primitive response, can increase the heart rate and myocardial workload and precipitate ventricular ectopics. The ectopics may eventually convert into VF or VT. For those who develop these rhythms, the loss of a regular cardiac output will accelerate myocardial ischaemia, metabolic acidosis, tissue hypoxia, acute underperfusion of vital organs and sudden death. Only immediate defibrillation can reverse this process (Resuscitation Council UK 2000b). Other factors can also affect the outcomes of in-hospital resuscitation (as shown in Table 9.1).

Table 9.1 Factors affecting outcomes of in-hospital resuscitation.

There are a number of factors that have a bearing on successful in-hospital resuscitation.

- *Early recognition of VT and VF* – improved outcomes occur if these rhythms are detected promptly and defibrillation delivered within three minutes or sooner after their onset (Gwinnutt *et al*. 2000).
- *Time taken to deliver a shock* – statistics indicate that for every minute that elapses before defibrillation, between 7% and 10% of patients will die who might have otherwise been saved (Cobbe *et al*. 1991). The work of Valenzuela *et al*. (2000) confirms this. In a study of 90 patients whose collapse was witnessed, the survival rate was 74% when the first shock was delivered within three minutes or less following the arrest call. When the interval to defibrillation exceeded this period, survival fell to 49%.
- *Patient variables* – if the patient is less than 70 years of age and a return of spontaneous circulation occurs within three minutes or less, then survival from cardiac arrest is more likely (Gwinnutt *et al*. 2000).
- *Location of the arrest* – patients in general wards experience reduced survival outcomes following a cardiac arrest (Gwinnutt *et al*. 2000). But a number of studies suggest that the introduction of AEDs will enable healthcare staff in these areas to challenge this trend (Coady 1999, Soar & Mckay 1998, Spearpoint *et al*. 2000).

Arrhythmias may also be triggered as a result of:

- *Cardiac disorders* – hypoxia, hypothermia, electrolyte disorders, drug toxicity (digoxin), electrocution and any cause leading to hypoxaemia.
- *Airway obstruction* – laryngospasm, foreign bodies, vomit and loss of airway control as a result of damage to central nervous system (CNS).
- *Respiratory failure* – pulmonary oedema, acute asthma, decreased respiratory drive due to CNS changes and inadequate respiratory effort as a result of exhaustion or opioid abuse.

Factors that impact on a successful cardiac defibrillation
- Transthoracic impedance
- Energy requirements
- Biphasic waveform defibrillation

The aim of defibrillation is to interrupt the chaotic pattern of ventricular impulses and restore normal conduction across the heart by delivering a low electrical current (Harris 2002). Direct current (DC) defibrillation in the early stages of VF depolarises the whole of the myocardial muscle and conducting system. Post-shock myocardial cells will enter a period of recovery, reset themselves and allow the sinoatrial node to restore sinus rhythm activity and produce organised myocardial fibre contraction (Cooper *et al.* 1998, Harris 2002).

Transthoracic impedance

Transthoracic impedance (TTI) plays a part in the level of cardiac response to a defibrillatory shock. Transthoracic impedance is defined as the resistance to current flow through chest wall, lung tissue and myocardium; hence the greater the resistance, the less the flow of current (Cooper *et al.* 1998). There are a number of practical means by which TTI can be reduced.

- Phase of respiration – shocks should be delivered at the end of expiration when there is less air in the lungs, thus reducing the distance between electrodes and heart. Patients should be disconnected from the ventilator or bagging circuit during defibrillation (Deakin *et al.* 1998).
- Paddle pressure – paddles must be firmly pressed against the chest as this reduces TTI and will ensure good contact; 10–12 kg of pressure per paddle should be applied (Resuscitation Council UK 2000a).
- Paddle surface area – increased paddle size lowers impedance (Jevon 2002).
- Defibrillation gel pads – protect skin from superficial burns, help to reduce impedance between pads and skin and enhance conduction. These should be replaced after 3–6 shocks or if they appear dry (Inwood & Cull 1997).
- Interval between shocks – impedance is reduced if shocks are delivered in close succession (Cooper *et al.* 1998). The first three shocks in the unresponsive patient should be given within 45 seconds.
- Positioning of paddles – it is important to ensure that the paddles are placed correctly (Heames *et al.* 2001, Mattei *et al.* 2002) as this facilitates maximal depolarisation of a critical mass of myocardium.

—*Apex–anterior position* – is the commonly used paddle placement for defibrillation and cardioversion. The 'sternal' paddle is placed to the right of the sternum, below the right clavicle. The 'apex' paddle must lie to the left of the chest, level with the fifth intercostal space in the zone of V_5 and V_6 (see Figures 9.1 and 9.2a).

—*Anterior–posterior position* – this approach is not easy, particularly if the patient is large. It should only be used when defibrillation with standard paddle technique has been ineffective or if the patient has a internal pacemaker or cardiac defibrillator. The patient must be placed on their right side. The anterior pad should be placed to the left of the sternal border and the posterior pad should be situated just below the left scapula.

—*Under breast/lateral to breast* – applicable when defibrillating women with large breasts. Pagan-Carlo *et al*. (1996) suggest that placement of the apex paddle under the breast or left lateral to the breast is preferable as it helps decrease thoracic impedance and raises current flow (as shown in Figure 9.2b). Paddles must never be placed over a nipple, clavicle or sternum or below the bottom rib.

—*Special considerations* – for patients with a left-sided internal pacemaker, the paddles should be at least 12–15 cm away from the unit (Resuscitation Council UK 2000a). If pacemaker is on the right, adopt the anterior–posterior position.

Energy requirements

The current standard practice for initial shock energy levels is 200 J, followed by a further 200 J. If there is no response, subsequent shocks should be at 360 J. However, should there be an episode of spontaneous circulation followed by a recurrence of VT/VF, then defibrillation should recommence with 200 J (see Chapter 6). It is important to deliver the shocks within 30–45 sec; this is possible with modern defibrillators as they recharge rapidly. The introduction of biphasic waveforms allows for energies of less than 200 J to be used which produce equal outcomes as standard monophasic waveforms that are typical of manual defibrillators (Wanchun *et al*. 2000).

Sternal gel pad (must be below
the right clavicle)

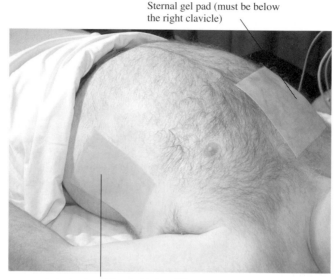

Apical gel pad (located below 5th
intercostal rib to the left of the thorax)

Fig. 9.1 Positioning of defibrillation gel pads.

Biphasic waveform defibrillation

Defibrillation waveform mapping has attracted much attention since the advent of internal cardiac defibrillators (ICD). The two most commonly described are 'monophasic' and 'biphasic' waveforms which are shaped by how they are generated and TTI.

- Currents that flow in one direction between electrodes over a specific period are referred to as *monophasic* and are generated by stored energy being discharged from a capacitor through the chest. Monophasic waveforms tend to be characterised by an initial positive upstroke representing the discharged energy or current. The appearance of the waveform changes when it reaches its peak level, decreasing gradually until it stops suddenly back at zero.

- *Biphasic* waveforms provide bidirectional flow of current in two phases, over a period of time, at a much lower energy than conventional defibrillators. The shape of the waveform is identical to a monophasic waveform but once the first phase is complete, the current then reverses and flows in a negative direction for the same period and stops abruptly (Faddy *et al*. 2003, Harris 2002, Tang *et al*. 2000).

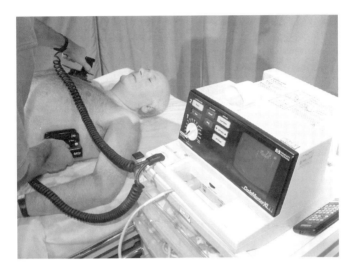

Fig. 9.2a Apex–anterior paddle position.

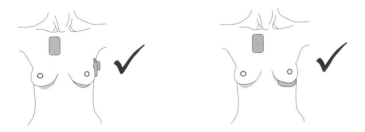

Fig. 9.2b Underbreast and lateral-to-breast paddle positions (adapted from Pagan-Carlo *et al.* 1996).

A meta-analysis investigating the advantage of integrating biphasic waveform technology into defibrillators concluded that at lower energies, biphasic defibrillators were as efficacious at terminating VF as standard 200 J monophasic waveforms (Faddy *et al.* 2003). Biphasic defibrillators were also more successful when compared to the use of consecutive escalating monophasic defibrillatory shocks. The benefits of lower energy levels include:

- early restoration of spontaneous circulation;
- reduced myocardial injury;
- decreased signs of ST segment elevation;
- potential hazards can be reduced.

At present there is no agreement on the ideal energy levels for biphasic waveform defibrillators (Jevon 2002).

OPERATING A MANUAL DEFIBRILLATOR

Manual defibrillators have been widely used to reverse VF or pulseless VT but have been confined to critical care settings. A typical device (as shown in Figure 9.3) comprises the following features, which may vary according to the manufacturer.

(1) On/off dial.
(2) Dial to select energy required.
(3) Charge button – this may also be found on paddles.
(4) Button for selecting the monitoring of the ECG trace through leads only.
(5) Button to increase amplitude of ECG trace.
(6) Switch for setting upper/lower alarm limits.
(7) Cardiac monitor.
(8) Modern defibrillators also have a synchronise mode that is activated by a switch or button. This is *only* selected for cardioversion of atrial and ventricular tachycardias (see later in the chapter).

Defibrillators also include an ECG cable, which permits monitoring of the cardiac rhythm. Most modern devices are also able to print a continuous rhythm strip and produce a record of the sequence of defibrillator shocks administered. All this activity can also be stored in the memory. Two other electrical cords leave the defibrillator and connect to an apex and a sternal paddle that are between 10 and 13 cm in diameter for the adult patient. When the power is on, pressing the paddles against the patient's chest will display the cardiac rhythm; in the arrest situation, this saves valuable time should the patient require defibrillation (see Figure 9.4). If the patient does not require defibrillation, the ECG leads may then be attached.

Paddle design may vary so knowledge of local equipment is vital. Figure 9.4 illustrates the function of various buttons in this model.

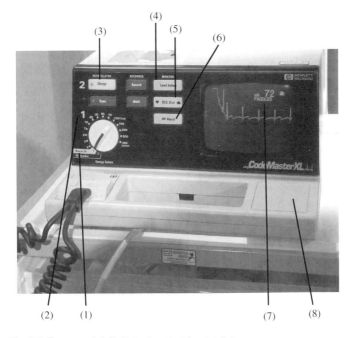

Fig. 9.3 The manual defibrillator (see text for details).

(1) The sternal paddle is for selecting the energy levels (on some models).
(2) The apex paddle is the charge button and is activated when depressed (on some models); this must be while the paddles are on the patient's chest.
(3) To deliver a shock, both discharge buttons must be depressed simultaneously.

Familiarity with the equipment is important and testing of the device should be carried out daily. Only persons who have been certified as competent must operate manual defibrillators. Table 9.2 provides a simplified procedure for performing manual defibrillation.

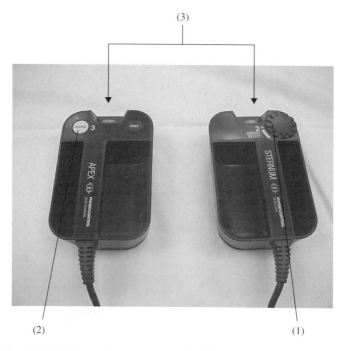

Fig. 9.4 Defibrillator paddles (see text for details).

Table 9.2 Procedure for performing manual defibrillation.

The following sequence has been adapted from the Resuscitation Council UK (2000a) guidelines in manual defibrillation.

- Confirm that patient has arrested and that cardiac arrest team or similar have been alerted.
- Place defibrillation gel pads on patient's thorax as recommended.
- Use defibrillation paddles to verify that the ECG rhythm is VF/VT as demonstrated in Figure 9.2a.
- If VT/VF is confirmed, 200 J must be selected with dial.
- The paddles must then be firmly applied onto the defibrillation gel pads.
- Once the 'charge' button on the paddles has been depressed, give a clear and loud verbal warning to 'stand clear'.
- Perform a comprehensive visual scan to ensure that all personnel and self are at safe distance away.
- Review the screen to confirm that the ECG is still displaying VF/VT.
- If satisfied, simultaneously press both discharge buttons to deliver the prescribed energy shock. If VF persists, continue shocking according to algorithm guidelines; proceed then to confirm and monitor the cardiac rhythm through the ECG leads (Bradbury *et al.* 2000).

Limitations of manual defibrillators

- They are heavy and bulky.
- Operation requires additional training to achieve competence.
- Without practice, skill in operating a manual defibrillator and rhythm interpretation declines. Keeping updated requires time away from wards (Moule & Albarran 2002).
- Use has been confined to critical care settings, by authorised staff only.

OPERATING AN AUTOMATED EXTERNAL DEFIBRILLATOR (AED)

The introduction of modern AEDs has overcome many of the obstacles associated with using manual defibrillators. Their ease of operation and safety features have meant that a broad range of first responders and rescuers are able to defibrillate without delay. Additionally, as the AED is programmed to assess the rhythm, the operator is not required to recognise or interpret cardiac arrhythmias. Due to these facilities, airline staff, paramedics and lay people with minimal training have been observed operating an AED promptly and efficiently (Capucci *et al.* 2002, Eames *et al.* 2003, Gottschalk *et al.* 2002, Page *et al.* 2000, Ross *et al.* 2001). Consequently there have been recommendations that all healthcare staff should be trained to use an AED to reduce unnecessary delays to vital life-saving treatment.

Shock advisory defibrillators

Following confirmation that the patient is not breathing and has no pulse, the rescuer must switch the AED on, attach the adhesive electrodes in the correct position and connect the cable to the patient (see Figures 9.5a–d). The machine will advise the rescuer to push the ANALYZE button (see Figure 9.6a). In some models electrographic analysis is automatic. The defibrillator will then proceed to evaluate whether or not the patient is in a shockable rhythm. To prevent artefactual errors that may contribute to unwanted delays, it is important that no one is touching the patient. The defibrillator may interpret VF or VT as artefact so it is vital that cardiac arrest is confirmed prior to attaching the pads and switching on the AED.

Should defibrillation be indicated, the AED will charge itself automatically to a predetermined level. During this period, all personnel should stand clear from the patient and avoid physical contact. When advised to defibrillate the patient, the operator should perform a visual check to ensure everyone has stepped away, after which the SHOCK button(s) must be pressed downwards (Figure 9.6b). Once the patient has been defibrillated, the rhythm must be reviewed by pushing the ANALYZE button and if the patient remains in VF or pulseless VT, up to three shocks may be delivered. If these are unsuccessful CPR must be started according to guidelines (see Chapter 6).

Many modern AEDs employ biphasic escalating (or non-escalating) waveform shocks and are programmed to deliver preset shocks in groups of three that are sufficient to terminate VF/VT in adult patients as recommended by guidelines (Liddle *et al.* 2003). Finally, as a result of the software, it is possible to obtain a full report of the patient's cardiac rhythm, a diagnosis of shockable rhythm and frequency of shocks administered (Cooper *et al.* 1998, Jevon 2002).

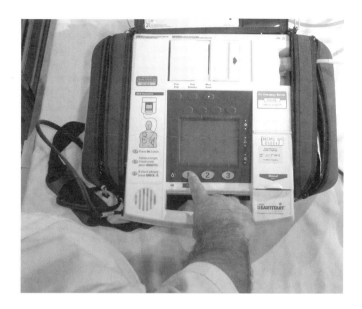

Fig. 9.5a Switching the AED on.

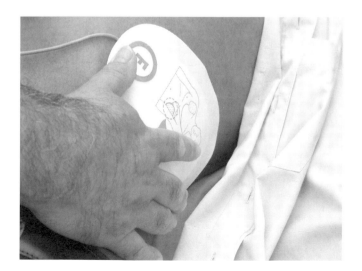

Fig. 9.5b Positioning of apical electrode.

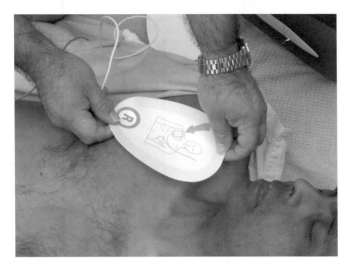

Fig. 9.5c Positioning of sternal electrode.

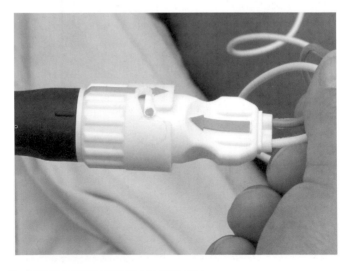

Fig. 9.5d Connecting electrodes to AED cable.

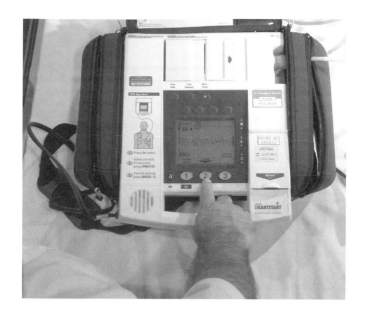

Fig. 9.6a Analysis of rhythm.

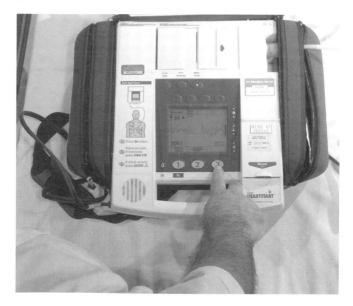

Fig. 9.6b Preparing to defibrillate the patient.

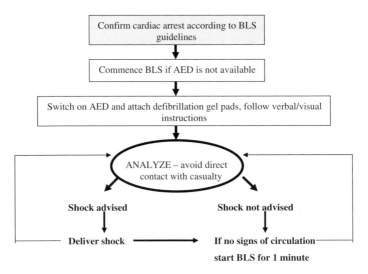

Fig. 9.7 Proposed revisions for AED algorithm (adapted from Jevon *et al*. 2003).

Although algorithms have been issued to guide operators of AEDs, Jevon *et al*. (2003) have proposed some minor improvements that could be incorporated to enhance and facilitate use; these are described in Figure 9.7.

SYNCHRONISED CARDIOVERSION

Defibrillators are also used to transform tachyarrhythmias of an atrial or ventricular origin into sinus rhythm, by selecting the synchronised cardioversion mode. Reasons for emergency cardioversion include:

- persistent atrial fibrillation/flutter;
- poor response or undesirable side-effects from drug therapy;
- patient has become haemodynamically unstable due to a tachyarrhythmia;
- sustained supraventricular tachycardias which produce signs of cardiovascular distress (Trohman & Parillo 2000).

The aim of electrical cardioversion is to depolarise the myocardium, interrupt the tachyarrhythmia and so enable the sinoatrial node to regain control with a sinus rhythm. While the techniques and safety procedures for delivering the shock are similar in most respects, there are four major differences between defibrillation and cardioversion:

- use of anaesthesia;
- synchronisation mode;
- selection of energy levels;
- complications.

Use of anaesthesia
Synchronised cardioversion is usually a planned treatment and the patient's consent is required. Patients are starved for at least four hours and given a short-acting anaesthetic. Anaesthetic support must be present.

Synchronisation mode
For this procedure, ECG monitoring and all the essential equipment for managing CPR must be available. Once the patient has been attached to the monitor and the trace is on screen, the 'synch' button must be activated. To verify this, the ECG should display bright synchronising signals/marks over the R waves. This ensures that the shock is triggered to take place on the R wave and not the T wave, as this might induce VF (Bennett 2002). Prior to the shock, the operator must check that only the R waves are synchronised. If the complexes are small, increase the amplitude. Operators need to be aware of the delay between the time the discharge buttons were depressed and the actual shock; this is because the defibrillator is detecting a shockable R wave. Hence the paddles must remain pressed firmly on the patient's chest and buttons depressed until the shock has been delivered. Some defibrillators default to unsynchronised mode after each shock. In others the 'synch' button must be switched off.

Energy levels
With cardioversion the delivery of energy levels may be low initially, but vary according to underlying rhythm. Recommended

shock energy levels for cardioversion are currently 100J, 200J and 360J (de Latorre *et al.* 2001).

Complications

- Systemic/cerebral embolism (with atrial fibrillation)
- Ventricular fibrillation
- Transient rhythm disturbances

Following the procedure, the patient must be placed in the recovery position until they regain consciousness. If the patient complains of residual chest pain, assess location, radiation, quality and intensity and administer prescribed analgesia accordingly.

OPERATING A DEFIBRILLATOR SAFELY

A number of safety issues are associated with operating a defibrillator, regardless of whether it is a manual device or an AED.

Casualty related

- GTN patches are explosive and should be removed prior to defibrillation; transdermal patches or ointments may redirect energy away from the heart.
- If the patient has a pacemaker, the relevant paddle should be placed at least 12–15cm from the device (Resuscitation Council UK 2000a).
- Ensure that there is no direct contact between defibrillation paddles and external pacing wires. Body jewellery, metal objects and medallions must be removed from the chest (Liddle *et al.* 2003).

External considerations

- Petrochemicals or inflammable spirits or fumes can ignite with a spark so remove casualty to a safe area, if necessary.
- Oxygen may need to be removed or switched off temporarily during defibrillation (Liddle *et al.* 2003) unless it is being delivered by a closed system.
- If the casualty is lying on a wet floor, covered in blood or soaked in rain, they should be removed to a safe and dry area.

The chest should be dried of any form of fluid that may conduct a shock.

Operator considerations

- The operator's hands must be kept dry.
- Use of gel pads minimises the risk of burns to the casualty; these should be replaced according to guidelines.
- Failure to keep paddles firmly pressed on the casualty's chest during shock delivery may result in flash arc.
- Paddles should only be charged either when on the casualty's chest (ideal option) or in their containers.
- Once defibrillation shocks have ended, the paddles must be replaced into their appropriate containers.
- The safety of bystanders and other staff is the responsibility of the person using the defibrillator. An audible verbal warning to all personnel to 'Stand clear' must be given by the operator.
- The operator must always perform a visual scan to ensure that nobody is directly or indirectly in contact with the casualty. Possible areas of indirect contact include any area of the bedframe, infusion stands, electric cables and intravenous infusions.

IMPLANTABLE CARDIAC DEFIBRILLATORS

A number of international trials have concluded that implantable cardiac defibrillators (ICDs) provide superior survival outcomes when compared to traditional pharmacological interventions for specific patients who are at risk of sudden cardiac death from ventricular dysrhythmias (AVID Investigators 1997, Moss *et al.* 1996, 2002, Trappe *et al.* 1997).

ICDs are implanted subcutaneously via the transvenous route in the left or right deltopectoral area, similar to a permanent pacemaker (Houghton & Kaye 2003, Porterfield *et al.* 1999). The procedure can be undertaken using local anaesthesia and intravenous sedation. An ICD comprises a generator (containing microprocessors, integrated circuits, memory boards and battery) plus one or more leads for pacing and defibrillation electrodes (Di Marco 2003). The software co-ordinates, senses, interprets, stores data and links with the different subsections of the system to provide an appropriate response (Pinski 2000). Current indications and guidelines for use are divided into primary and secondary prevention.

For primary prevention:

- non-sustained VT;
- inducible VT on electrophysiological testing;
- myocardial infarction, depressed left ventricular function with an ejection fraction (EF) of 35% or less (normal ejection fraction 65–70%);
- high risk of sudden death due to familial cardiac conditions: long QT syndrome or arrhythmogenic right ventricular dysplasia.

For secondary prevention:

- survivors of cardiac arrest due to either VT or VF;
- spontaneous sustained VT associated with symptomatic haemodynamic compromise;
- sustained VT without causing syncope or a cardiac arrest in highly symptomatic patients who have an associated reduced EF (<35%) but whose heart failure is not totally debilitating (Houghton & Kaye 2003).

Modern ICDs are highly sophisticated, with a battery that may last anything from five to nine years, and can be programmed to perform multiple tasks including:

- record intracardiac electrograms, allowing review of episodes of rhythm disturbances and defibrillation;
- arrhythmia detection;
- delivery of high-energy unsynchronised defibrillation shocks;
- discharge low-energy synchronised shocks (cardioversion) for VT;
- delivery of low- and high-energy shocks (tiered therapy);
- antitachycardia pacing;
- back-up pacing for bradyarrhythmias (Di Marco 2003, Pinski 2000)

Worldwide, the number of patients having these devices fitted is increasing annually (Garratt 1998, Tagney 2003). It is important to know how to manage such individuals should the ICD fail or if defibrillation is required. Current guidelines suggest that paddles should be positioned at least 10–12 cm from the device. Shocks will not damage the equipment but it is advisable that the ICD should be deactivated to avoid the device potentially inducing VT or VF (Pinski 2000).

REVIEW OF LEARNING

❏ Early defibrillation improves survival outcomes following a cardiac arrest.
❏ Healthcare professionals must be skilled in recognising a cardiac arrest and know how to respond effectively.
❏ Intervention with rapid defibrillation is an emergency procedure that must be delivered promptly, effectively and safely.
❏ The types of defibrillators currently available include manual, automatic and semiautomatic.
❏ In the event of a cardiac arrest, if a defibrillator is not immediately available, CPR should be started.
❏ Factors impacting on successful cardiac defibrillation include transthoracic impedance, energy requirements, biphasic waveform defibrillation and the effects of drugs.
❏ The paddles must stay on the casualty's chest between shocks as this reduces delays to defibrillation.
❏ Any healthcare professional responsible for performing BLS must be competent in using an AED and must update regularly.
❏ Synchronised cardioversion is usually an elective procedure used to transform tachyarrhythmias of an atrial or ventricular origin into sinus rhythm.
❏ During cardioversion it is vital that the 'synch' button is activated. Verification involves checking that the cardiac monitor displays bright synchronising signals/marks over the R waves.
❏ Staff operating a defibrillator must always be aware of the potential dangers and hazards that may occur to the patient and bystanders while delivering a shock.

Case study

You are working a night shift and decide to get a snack from the vending machine. You arrive at your destination and hear a noise. Slumped on a chair, you find a gentleman who is unrousable and whose shirt is soaked in coffee. **What do you do next?** Write down what you might do.

You confirm that the patient has arrested and assess for signs of respiration and circulation. If these are absent, get immediate assistance from the nearest ward or telephone, giving the exact location. Return to the casualty and place him in a position to begin basic life support. Use the head tilt, chin lift manoeuvre to open the airway and assess that it is patent.

The AED arrives almost immediately and you switch it on. You remove the casualty's shirt and note that he is wearing a long gold chain. Write down what you would do next.

Remove all jewellery and metal. Dry the casualty's chest as much as possible. Place the sternal gel pad below the right clavicle and the other gel pad lateral to the left nipple with the top of the pad 7 cm below the axilla. Connect the cable to the AED.

What is your next action?

Follow voice and visual directions on the AED. The device instructs you to press the ANALYZE button but first make sure that nobody is touching the casualty. Within seconds, the AED confirms that the casualty is in a shockable rhythm. The voice prompt will then warn all personnel to stand clear. In the meantime, the AED will charge to a pre-set level; you may see this on the screen or hear an audible sound. You will then be advised to press the shock button(s). Before doing so, check your environment and make sure everyone has stepped back and that it is safe to defibrillate the patient. Once the patient has been shocked, reanalyse the rhythm. If the patient is still in VF follow the ALS algorithm (in Chapter 6).

The second shock has been successful, as evident by ECG analysis. **What would you do next?**

Continued

Check the airway then assess for signs of breathing and the carotid pulse for signs of circulation. If the casualty is stable then arrange for transfer to the coronary care unit. During transfer, monitor the ECG, non-invasive blood pressure and oxygen saturation (see Chapter 12). Provide an accurate handover and document all relevant actions/ interventions during the arrest and ensure the next of kin are notified.

CONCLUSION

Being a healthcare professional carries many responsibilities and the maintenance of competence in performing BLS and use of an AED can be regarded as one realistic expectation. Early defibrillation has been established as a major component of the Chain of Survival which, when administered promptly and safely, can have a positive and significant impact on patient outcomes. With newer devices being developed that are easy to use and safer, the scope for improving survival rates from cardiac arrest will increase. However, the challenge for all healthcare professionals is to keep updated and have the opportunity to practise regularly in order to be able to recognise and respond to a cardiac arrest call effectively.

REFERENCES

American Heart Association and International Liaison Committee on Resuscitation (2000) Adult basic life support. *Resuscitation* **46** (1–3), 29–71.

AVID Investigators (1997) A comparison of anti-arrhythmic therapy with implantable defibrillators in patients resuscitated from near fatal arrhythmias. *New England Journal of Medicine* **337**, 1576–83.

Bennett, D.H. (2002) *Cardiac Arrhythmias: Practical Notes on Interpretation and Treatment*, 6th edn. Arnold, London.

Bossaert, L., Handley, A., Marsden, A. *et al*. (1998) European Resuscitation Council guidelines for the use of automated external defibrillators by EMS providers and first responders. *Resuscitation* **37** (2), 91–4.

Bradbury, N., Hyde, D. & Nolan, J. (2000) Reliability of the ECG monitoring with gel/paddle combination after defibrillation. *Resuscitation* **44**, 203–6.

Capucci, A., Ascheri, D., Pieploi, M.F., Bardy, G., Iconomu, E. & Arverdi, M. (2002) Tripling survival from sudden cardiac arrest via early defibrillation without traditional education in cardiopulmonary resuscitation. *Circulation* **106**, 1065–70.

Coady, E. (1999) A strategy for nurse defibrillation in general wards. *Resuscitation* **42**, 183–6.

Cobbe, S., Redmond, M., Watson, J., Hollingworth, J. & Carrington, D.J. (1991) 'Heartstart Scotland' – initial experience of a national scheme for out of hospital defibrillation. *British Medical Journal* **302**, 1517–20.

Cooper, M., More, J., Robb, A. & Ness, V. (1998) A guide to defibrillation. *Emergency Nurse* **6** (3), 16–21.

Deakin, C.D., McLaren, R.M., Petley, G.W., Clewlow, F. & Darymple-Hay, M.J. (1998) Effects of positive end-expiratory pressure on transthoracic impedance – implications for defibrillation. *Resuscitation* **37**, 9–12.

de Latorre, F., Nolan, J., Robertson, C., Chamberlain, D. & Basketl, P. (2001) ERC guidelines 2000 for adult Advanced Life Support. *Resuscitation* **48**, 211–21.

Di Marco, J.P. (2003) Implantable cardioverter-defibrillators. *New England Journal of Medicine* **349** (19), 1836–47.

Eames, P., Larsen, P.D. & Galletly, D.C. (2003) Comparison of ease of use of three automated defibrillators by untrained people. *Resuscitation* **58**, 25–30.

Faddy, S.C., Powell, J. & Craig, J. (2003) Biphasic and monophasic shocks for transthoracic defibrillation: a meta-analysis of randomised controlled trials. *Resuscitation* **58** (1), 9–16.

Garratt, C.J. (1998) A new evidence base for implantable defibrillator therapy. *European Heart Journal* **19**, 189–91.

Gottschalk, A., Burmeister, M.A., Freitag, M., Cavus, E. & Standl, T. (2002) Influence of early defibrillation on the survival rate and quality of life after CPR in prehospital emergency medical service in a Gerrman metropolitan area. *Resuscitation* **53**, 15–20.

Gwinnutt, C., Coulumbo, M. & Harris, R. (2000) Outcome after cardiac arrest in adults in UK hospitals: effect of the 1997 guidelines. *Resuscitation* **47**, 125–35.

Harris, J. (2002) Biphasic defibrillation. *Emergency Nurse* **10** (7), 33–7.

Heames, R., Sado, D. & Deakin, C.D. (2001) Do doctors position defibrillator paddles correctly? Observational study. *British Medical Journal* **322**, 1393–4.

Holmberg, M., Holmberg, S. & Herlitz, J. (2000) Incidence, duration and survival of ventricular fibrillation in out of hospital cardiac patients arrests in Sweden. *Resuscitation* **44** (1), 7–17.

Houghton, T. & Kaye, G.C. (2003) Implantable devices for treating tachyarrhythmias. *British Medical Journal* **327**, 333–6.

Inwood, H. & Cull, C. (1997) Defibrillation. *Professional Nurse* **13** (3), 165–8.

Jevon, P. (2002) *Advanced Cardiac Life Support: A Practical Guide.* Butterworth Heinemann, Oxford.

Jevon, P., Walton, E. & Baldock, C. (2003) AED algorithm: suggestions for improvement. *British Journal of Resuscitation* **2** (1), 11–12.

Liddle, R., Davies, C.S., Colquhoun, M. & Handley, A.J. (2003) ABC of resuscitation: the automated external defibrillator. *British Medical Journal* **327**, 1216–18.

Mattei, L., Mckay, U., Lepper, M.W. & Soar, J. (2002) Do nurses and physiotherapists require training to use an automated external defibrillator? *Resuscitation* **53**, 277–80.

Moss, A., Jackson, W., Cannom, D. *et al.* (1996) Improved survival with an implanted defibrillator in patients with coronary disease at high risk for ventricular arrhythmia. Multicentre Automatic Defibrillator Trial. *New England Journal of Medicine* **335** (26), 1993–40.

Moss, A., Zareba, W., Hall, W.J. *et al.* (2002) Prophylactic implantation of a defibrillator in patients with myocardial infarction and reduced ejection fraction. *New England Journal of Medicine* **346**, 877–83.

Moule, P. & Albarran, J.W. (2002) Automated external defibrillation as part of BLS: implications for education and practice. *Resuscitation* **54**, 333–70.

Pagan-Carlo, L.A., Spencer, K., Robertson, C., Dengler, A., Birkett, C., & Kerber, R.E. (1996) Thoracic defibrillation: importance of avoiding electrode placement directly on the breast. *Journal of the American College of Cardiology* **27**, 449–52.

Page, J., Kowal, R., Zagrodsky, J. *et al.* (2000) Use of automated external defibrillators by a US airline. *New England Journal of Medicine* **343** (17), 1210–16.

Pinski, S.L. (2000) Emergencies related to implantable cardioverter-defibrillators. *Critical Care Medicine* **28** (10)(suppl), N174–180.

Porterfield, L., Gonce Morton, P. & Butze, E. (1999) The evolution of internal defibrillators. *Critical Care Clinics of North America* **11** (3), 303–10.

Resuscitation Council UK (2000a) *Advanced Life Support Provider Manual*, 4th edn. Resuscitation Council UK, London.

Resuscitation Council UK (2000b) *Guidelines for the Use of Automated External Defibrillators: Resuscitation Guidelines*. Resuscitation Council UK, London.

Ross, P., Nolan, J., Hill, E., Dawson, J., Whimser, F. & Skinner, D. (2001) The use of AEDs by police officers in the city of London. *Resuscitation* **50**, 141–6.

Soar, J. & Mckay, U. (1998) A revised role for the hospital cardiac arrest team? *Resuscitation* **38**, 145–9.

Spearpoint, K., McLean, C. & Zidemann, D. (2000) Early defibrillation and the chain of survival in 'in-hospital' adult cardiac arrest: minutes count. *Resuscitation* **44**, 165–9.

Tagney, J. (2003) Implantable cardioverter defibrillators: developing evidence-based care. *Nursing Standard* **17** (16), 33–6.

Tang, W., Weil, M.H. & Sun, S. (2000) Low-energy biphasic waveform defibrillation reduces the severity of post resuscitation myocardial dysfunction. *Critical Care Medicine* **28** (11)(suppl), N222–4.

Trappe, H.-J., Wenzlaff, P., Pfitzner, P. & Fieguth, H.-G. (1997) Long-term follow-up of patients with implantable cardioverter defibrillators and mild, moderate or severe impairment of left ventricular impairment. *Heart* **78**, 243–49.

Trohman, R.G. & Parillo, J.E. (2000) Direct current cardioversion: indications, techniques and recent advances. *Critical Care Medicine* **28** (10)(suppl), N170–73.

Valenzuela, T.D., Roe, D., Nichol, G., Clark, L., Spaite, D. & Hardman, R. (2000) Outcomes of rapid defibrillation by security officers after cardiac arrest in casinos. *New England Journal of Medicine* **343** (17), 1206–9.

Drugs and Delivery

10

INTRODUCTION

The most important intervention in successful resuscitation is defibrillation and nothing should delay this. Where defibrillation has failed to restore circulation for ventricular fibrillation (VF) or pulseless ventricular tachycardia (VT), and where it is not indicated, there are a number of drugs that may be given to support or improve myocardial performance. Three of these, adrenaline/epinephrine, atropine and amiodarone, are currently included within the advanced life support (ALS) universal algorithm. Other drugs may be given for specific indications before, during and after cardiac arrest. Even if few drugs are supported by strong evidence (Baskett 2000), the body of research is growing (Lockey & Nolan 2001, Madrid & Sendlebach 2001). Given the increasingly international collaboration in this field, American names for drugs are often employed. *Epinephrine* is the term for adrenaline and *lidocaine* is used for lignocaine.

AIMS

This chapter reviews the drugs most commonly used during advanced resuscitation, including dosage and modes of delivery.

LEARNING OUTCOMES

At the end of the chapter the reader should be able to:

- ❏ identify the *routes available for the administration of drugs* for resuscitation;
- ❏ discuss the *advantages and disadvantages* of alternative routes;
- ❏ describe the *mode of action* of the first-line drugs used in resuscitation;

❏ describe the *role of healthcare professionals* in administering drugs during a resuscitation attempt;
❏ state the *indications, contraindications and dosages* of other resuscitation drugs.

ROUTES OF ADMINISTRATION

During resuscitation, drugs may be administered to the adult by a number of routes:

• peripheral intravenous
• central venous
• tracheal.

Direct intracardiac administration of drugs is not recommended.

Peripheral cannulation

Where intravenous (IV) access has been established prior to cardiac arrest, the *in situ* cannula should be used. Where a patient has developed chest pain or has become acutely unwell, inserting a cannula should be performed at the earliest opportunity, not least because it will be needed to administer adequate analgesia.

Peripheral cannulation is a skill that is currently performed by nurses and other healthcare professionals. However, inserting a peripheral cannula during a resuscitation attempt is not easy, because the patient's arms move with the motion of chest compressions and peripheral veins collapse because of poor cardiac output. The usual advice to cannulate as peripherally as possible should be reversed; the largest available veins should be cannulated, most commonly in the antecubital fossa. If possible, a sample of blood should be withdrawn while cannulating and care should be taken with the disposal of sharps.

If the cannula is patent, drugs can be given through it at any time other than during defibrillation. All drugs should be flushed with 20 ml of normal saline and if possible, the arm should be raised. Without these manoeuvres, the drug will remain in the peripheral circulation. It has been suggested that it takes up to five minutes for a drug administered by a peripheral cannula during cardiopulmonary resuscitation (CPR) to reach the heart and the central circulation (Resuscitation Council UK 2000).

Central venous cannulation
Two routes are commonly used:

- internal jugular veins
- subclavian veins.

For routine placement, the preferred site is the subclavian vein (EPIC Project 2001) but during resuscitation, the internal jugular vein is often preferred (Polderman & Girbes 2002). In most cases the Seldinger technique is used (Hinds & Watson 1996):

- the vein is punctured with a needle and syringe;
- a wire is passed through the needle into the vein;
- the needle is withdrawn;
- the cannula is passed over the wire into the vein;
- the wire is removed, leaving the cannula in the vein.

Early complications of the procedure include injury during insertion, pneumothorax and air embolus (Woodrow 2002).

Tracheal administration of drugs
This technique requires the presence of an endotracheal or tracheostomy tube. Only certain drugs can be given via this route (see Table 10.1). There are doubts as to whether the administration of drugs via the endotracheal (ET) tube is beneficial for out-of-hospital arrests (Niemann & Stratton 2000, Niemann et al. 2002). There have also been suggestions for higher dosages when giving drugs by this route (Manisterski et al. 2002). In the meantime, the recommendations (Resuscitation Council UK 2000) are that 2–3 times the dosage of the drug can be given via the ET tube, diluted to a volume of 10–20 ml. Drugs given via a laryngeal mask airway are not reliably absorbed and so this is not recommended (Prengel et al. 2001).

It has been recommended that the drugs should be diluted with sterile water, injected through a catheter placed distal to the end of the ET tube and then followed with quick ventilations to disperse the drug (Baskett 2000). However, this is time consuming and recent work suggests that simple instillation into the ET tube is as effective (Resuscitation Council UK 2000). This method also allows the use of pre-filled syringes. Twice the recommended dose for both adrenaline/epinephrine (2 mg) and atropine (6 mg), given during cardiac arrest, involve instilling 20 ml of solution.

DRUG ADMINISTRATION

Patient group directions (PGDs) allow nurses and other non-medical staff to give drugs before a patient has been seen by a doctor (DoH 2000). There is little evidence for extending PGDs to authorise nurses and others to administer cardiac arrest drugs in hospital, though some trusts utilise group directives to permit the administration of adrenaline/epinephrine for patients with acute anaphylaxis (NHSE North West 2003). Undertaking an advanced course in resuscitation does not automatically authorise nurses or other non-medical healthcare professionals to administer drugs during resuscitation without prescription. Practitioners should be aware of and be guided by local policies for the administration of drugs and infusions. The fact that the patient has suffered cardiac arrest should not compromise the usual standards for the administration of medicines as, in spite of the emergency situation, incorrect administration of drugs can make matters worse. The pre-filled syringes for different drugs may look similar and are of a standard size. The urgency of the situation and the need for a rapid response to a request for a drug should not excuse careful checking (Nursing and Midwifery Council 2002).

Table 10.1 Drugs and tracheal route (reprinted with permission from Resuscitation Council UK 2000).

Drugs that can be administered via the trachea	Drugs that cannot be administered via the trachea
Adrenaline/epinephrine Vasopressin Atropine Lignocaine (lidocaine) Naloxone	Calcium salts Sodium bicarbonate Amiodarone

Cardiac arrest trolleys must contain first-line drugs, ideally in the form of pre-filled syringes (see Chapter 3). There have been calls for a standardised format for drugs kits (Jowett *et al.* 2001) but in the absence of this, staff should familiarise themselves with the contents of drug boxes on cardiac arrest trolleys. There are two types of syringes in common usage.

Pre-filled syringes

As the name implies, these are simply syringes which are pre-filled with the drug in its standard dose and diluted appropriately. To administer the drug, the box has to be opened, the cap removed and then the drug is ready for injection (see Figure 10.1).

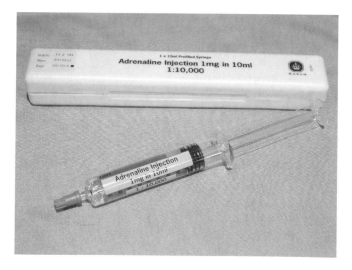

Fig. 10.1 Aurum pre-filled syringe.

Min-I-Jet

These syringes (as shown in Figure 10.2) require assembly immediately prior to drug administration. After emptying the components from the box, the yellow protective caps must be removed (as seen in Figure 10.3). The barrel and the plunger must then be screwed together (see Figure 10.4). After expelling the air, the syringe is ready for use (see Figure 10.5).

Many of the drug dosages in the prefilled syringes are standard, although this is not always the case. Practitioners should be aware that drugs come in different dosages.

Drug calculations

The dosages of resuscitation drugs are expressed in a number of ways and this can be confusing.

- Standard weight – for example, atropine 3 mg.
- Solution strength – this requires both a volume and a solution strength to be prescribed; for example, 50 ml of 8.4% sodium bicarbonate. Where a drug dose is expressed as a percentage, it means grams per 100 ml. So, for example, sodium bicarbonate 8.4% contains 8.4 g of sodium chloride in 100 ml of solution. Therefore a 50 ml dose contains 4.2 g of sodium bicarbonate.
- Dilution – this also requires both a dilution and a volume, e.g. adrenaline 10 ml of 1:10000. Where a drug is expressed as a dilution, it means grams in ml of solution. So, for example, adrenaline 1:10000 contains 1 gram in 10000 ml; that is, 1 mg in 10 ml.

All drug administration during cardiac arrest must be fully documented.

FIRST-LINE DRUGS

Adrenaline/epinephrine

Adrenaline/epinephrine is a naturally occurring substance that stimulates the sympathetic nervous system (SNS). The alpha-adrenergic effect of adrenaline causes arteriolar vasoconstriction, redirecting blood flow away from the peripheries to essential organs such as the heart and the brain. In addition, in a beating heart it increases myocardial contractility.

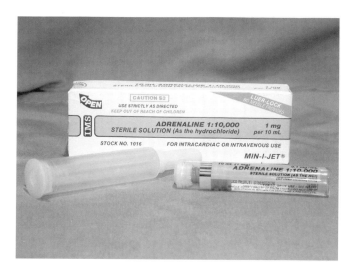

Fig. 10.2 Min-I-Jet assembly.

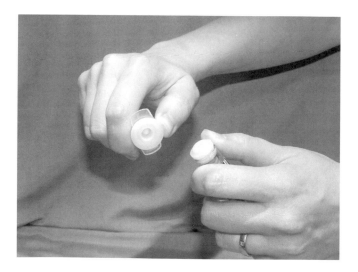

Fig. 10.3 Min-I-Jet assembly.

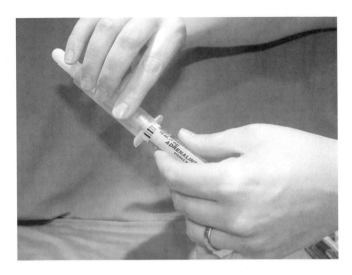

Fig. 10.4 Min-I-Jet assembly.

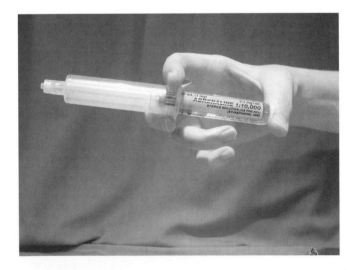

Fig. 10.5 Min-I-Jet assembly.

As the purpose is to improve cerebral and coronary blood flow during CPR, adrenaline/epinephrine can be administered on both sides of the universal algorithm. It achieves these changes by increasing peripheral vascular resistance and raising aortic diastolic pressure. The single exception to this is when a DC shock has terminated VF/VT into pulseless electrical activity (PEA). In this case, it is possible that the heart is beating but the cardiac output cannot be detected. This is known as myocardial stunning. Adrenaline/epinephrine is a powerful pro-arrhythmic and is very dangerous when given outside its limited indications (Johnstone *et al.* 2003). If it is given during this period, it can provoke further arrhythmias and so it should be withheld for the first minute of PEA after successful defibrillation. After a minute the pulse should be rechecked. If there is no pulse, CPR should be recommenced and adrenaline/epinephrine can be given safely.

Adrenaline/epinephrine for injection is supplied in two strengths: 1:1000 and 1:10000. The concentrations are therefore 1 mg/ml and 0.1 mg/ml The dose in cardiac arrest is 1 mg every three minutes. This is usually given by pre-filled syringe as 10 ml of 1:10000 solution.

Larger dosages of adrenaline/epinephrine are no longer recommended.

- A smaller dose of 500 µg can be given intramuscularly in severe anaphylaxis. This may be given as 0.5 ml of 1:1000 solution.
- An infusion of adrenaline/epinephrine of 2–10 µg per minute can be given to increase heart rate as an interim measure while awaiting transvenous pacing for symptomatic bradycardia.
- Unwanted effects include an increase in myocardial oxygen consumption and arrhythmias which may be further detrimental in the patient with cardiac ischaemia.
- Local protocols for the administration of adrenaline/epinephrine infusion should be consulted.

Atropine
Atropine blocks the action of acetylcholine at muscarinic receptors in the parasympathetic nervous system (PNS). Parasympa-

thetic stimulation via the vagus nerve slows the heart. Blocking this in the sinoatrial (SA) node increases automaticity and therefore heart rate. Blocking parasympathetic activity in the atrioventricular (AV) node facilitates conduction through the node.

- Atropine is given to increase heart rate.
- In symptomatic bradycardia, the dose is 500 µg repeated as necessary to a maximum dosage of 3 mg, the dose generally accepted to cause full parasympathetic blockade (Mader *et al.* 2000).
- A 3 mg dose via the IV route is recommended in asystole and pulseless electrical activity (PEA) of a rate below 60 bpm. This dose should only be given once.
- The evidence base for the use of atropine in cardiac arrest is sparse.

The role of the autonomic nervous system

There are two branches of the autonomic nervous system (ANS): the sympathetic (SNS) and the parasympathetic (PNS). The heart is supplied by both: by the vagus nerve from the PNS and the cardiac accelerator nerves from the SNS. Stimulation of the PNS slows the heart and reduces the force of contraction, while stimulation of the SNS has the opposite effect, speeding the heart and increasing the force of contraction. Depression of one half of the system produces similar results to stimulation of the other half (Hopkins 1999). In health the PNS is dominant, slowing the heart to its normal rate of about 70 beats per minute. In hearts that have no nervous supply (such as transplanted hearts), this 'parasympathetic brake' is absent and the resting heart rate is about 90–100 beats per minute (Lamb *et al.* 1991).

The side-effects of the drugs acting on the ANS (seen in Table 10.2) are related to the physiology of the organs supplied by its branches (Hinchliff *et al.* 1996, Hopkins 1999, Prosser *et al.* 2000).

Table 10.2 Effects of the autonomic nervous system.

Organ	Sympathetic stimulation (parasympathetic blockade)	Parasympathetic stimulation (sympathetic blockade)
Heart	Increased rate and contractility	Decreased rate and contractility
Blood vessels	Constriction	Dilation
Lungs	Bronchial dilation	Bronchial constriction
Eye	Pupils dilate	Pupils constrict

Amiodarone

Amiodarone is a complex drug, acting in many ways (Gonzalez *et al.* 1998). It works by increasing the duration of the action potential, though it also has antisympathetic and calcium channel-blocking properties (Taylor 2002). Amiodarone reduces membrane excitability and increases the refractory period, therefore making cardiac cells less susceptible to transmitting ectopic impulses.

A number of studies have shown the effectiveness of amiodarone during cardiac arrest. In the Amiodarone in Out-of-Hospital Resuscitation of Refractory Sustained Ventricular Tachycardia (ARREST) Trial (Kudenchuk *et al.* 1999), it proved better than placebo in terminating VF/VT. Similarly, the Amiodarone versus Lidocaine in Prehospital Ventricular Fibrillation Evaluation (ALIVE) (Dorian *et al.* 2002) reported improved results using amiodarone rather than lignocaine. Even if these trials did not demonstrate increased survival to discharge and beyond (Taylor 2002), there is sufficient evidence to recommend the use of amiodarone in VF/VT cardiac arrest if the initial three-shock sequence has been unsuccessful.

- Because of its unique pharmacological properties, amiodarone is effective in the management of both atrial and ventricular rhythms.
- The dosage given will depend on the situation and administration should preferably be via a central vein.
- After three unsuccessful defibrillator shocks for VF/VT cardiac arrest, 300 mg diluted in 5% dextrose up to a volume

of 20 ml should be administered after adrenaline/epinephrine. Pre-filled syringes are available.

- In the peri-arrest period, amiodarone is effective in both broad and narrow complex tachyarrhythmias. The dose is 150 mg delivered over ten minutes and repeated if necessary. Alternatively 300 mg can be given over one hour.

- The usual maximum daily dose of amiodarone is 1.2 g (British National Formulary 2003), but this can be increased up to 2 g (Resuscitation Council UK 2000).

- Intravenous infusion may be necessary and local policies should be consulted for these. It should be remembered that all antiarrhythmic drugs are also pro-arrhythmic.

- The major side-effects of amiodarone are hypotension and bradycardia.

OTHER DRUGS USED IN CARDIAC ARREST

Lignocaine/lidocaine

- Lignocaine/lidocaine is indicated for refractory VF/VT when the first three defibrillator shocks have failed to produce a return of spontaneous circulation and when amiodarone is unavailable.

- It acts by suppressing the excitability of ventricular cells.

- The initial dose in VF is 100 mg and in haemodynamically stable VT, 50 mg should be administered intravenously.

- An infusion may be necessary according to local protocols.

- Side-effects are drowsiness, confusion and convulsions.

Sodium bicarbonate

There has been considerable controversy over the use of sodium bicarbonate as a buffer to correct acidosis during cardiac arrest and there is little research to support its use (Bar-Joseph *et al.* 2002). Initial support for its routine use has diminished (Gazmuri 1999). Blood gas analysis is often unavailable quickly and in any case, arterial blood gases do not reflect intracellular values. In some cases, administration of sodium bicarbonate may worsen intracellular acidosis. Additionally, some degree of acidosis increases cerebral blood flow, so normalisation of values may hinder cerebral protection (Resuscitation Council UK 2000). However, acidosis reduces cardiac contractility (Adgey 1998) and so small dosages (50 mmol intravenously; 50 ml of 8.4% solution) can be given in the following circumstances.

- Severe acidosis – pH <7.1 or BE <−10. This may exist prior to the cardiac arrest.
- Cardiac arrest associated with hyperkalaemia (raised potassium levels).
- Cardiac arrest associated with tricyclic antidepressant (for example, dothiepin, imipramine) overdose.
- Sodium bicarbonate causes tissue damage if the cannula extravasates; a large vessel such as the external jugular vein is a preferred route for administration.
- A flush with 0.9% saline must follow sodium bicarbonate infusion.
- If given with calcium chloride, calcium carbonate is precipitated.
- The tracheal route must always be avoided.

Calcium chloride
Calcium is vital for myocardial contraction. A dose of 10 ml of 10% calcium chloride can be given in PEA for:

- hyperkalaemia (high potassium levels);
- hypocalcaemia (low calcium levels);
- overdose of calcium channel-blocking drugs (diltiazem, verapamil, nifedipine).

Intravenous calcium can cause severe tissue injury if extravasation occurs around the cannula.

Potassium chloride
- Hypokalaemia can cause tachyarrhythmias.
- If serum potassium is known to be low, potassium chloride up to 60 mmol at a maximum rate of 30 mmol per hour, appropriately diluted, can be administered.
- Concentrated solutions of potassium chloride are extremely dangerous and can make a poor situation worse.

Magnesium sulphate

- Low magnesium and low potassium levels can be associated and can cause tachyarrhythmias.
- Magnesium sulphate is indicated for refractory VF/VT where low magnesium is suspected and in torsade de pointes (polymorphic VT; see Chapter 8).
- The dose is 2.5 g over 1–2 minutes. This is generally given as 5 ml of 50% magnesium sulphate solution.

Adenosine

- Adenosine temporarily blocks conduction through the AV node. If a supraventricular tachycardia (usually narrow but wide if there is aberrance) involves re-entry within or through the AV node, adenosine can break the circuit, converting the arrhythmia to sinus rhythm. In the absence of a re-entry mechanism, adenosine stops the ventricles for a few seconds, allowing identification of an atrial arrhythmia.
- The period of ventricular standstill can be alarming for both staff and patient.
- Cardiac monitoring is mandatory and facilities for recording the ECG should be available.
- Side-effects are transient but unpleasant and include chest pain and hot flushes. Patients should be warned in advance.
- The dose is 3 mg, 6 mg, then 12 mg, repeated as necessary.
- Rapid administration followed by a large flush is necessary.

Naloxone

- Naloxone reverses the effects of opioid administration and is very effective in treatment of opioid overdose, both iatrogenic (caused by medical treatment) and through drug abuse.
- It should be readily available wherever opioids are given.
- The duration of action is shorter than for opioids so frequent administration or infusion may be necessary.
- The dose is 0.4–0.8 mg as required.

Esmolol

- Esmolol is a short-acting beta-blocker, which can be used for narrow complex tachycardias.
- Like all beta-blockers, it can cause bradycardia and left ventricular failure.

- The dose is 40 mg over one minute followed by an infusion, maximum 0.1 mg/kg/min.

Verapamil
- Verapamil is a calcium channel blocker, which can be effective in supraventricular tachycardia.
- It should not be given where the origin of the tachycardia is in doubt (i.e. wide complexes) or in conjunction with beta-blockers.
- It can cause bradycardia and hypotension.
- The dose is 5–10 mg over two minutes.

FUTURE PROSPECTS

Though the use of drugs in resuscitation has declined in the last decade (Baskett 2000), the evidence base for the use of drugs during cardiac arrest has grown. There has been much interest in the role of vasopressin rather than adrenaline/epinephrine to cause peripheral constriction (Krismer *et al.* 2001) though it is not yet recommended. Since the majority of cardiac arrests are associated with coronary artery disease, the use of thrombolytic drugs has been suggested and initial studies are promising (Bottiger & Martin 2001). Larger scale studies are anticipated (Nolan *et al.* 2002).

REVIEW OF LEARNING

❏ Defibrillation is the only proven treatment for ventricular fibrillation and nothing should delay it.
❏ However, if defibrillation is not indicated or unsuccessful, certain drugs may be given.
❏ Drugs should preferably be administered via an intravenous route. Some drugs can be given via an endotracheal tube.
❏ Adrenaline/epinephrine 1 mg is given every three minutes during cardiac arrest. Its purpose is to improve basic life support by directing the cardiac output to the heart and the brain.
❏ Atropine increases heart rate; 3 mg can be given for asystole or PEA rate less than 60.
❏ Amiodarone slows and stabilises the heart; 300 mg can be given after adrenaline/epinephrine in VF/VT if the first three shocks are unsuccessful.

❏ Other drugs can be given for specific indications.
❏ It is important to keep a record of all drugs and infusions administered during the arrest.

Case study

A patient suffers VF cardiac arrest and is defibrillated three times unsuccessfully. **What drugs may be considered immediately afterwards and how do they act?**

CPR should be commenced. To augment this by causing vasoconstriction, adrenaline/epinephrine should be given. If intravenous access is available, the dose is 1 mg, usually given as 10 ml of 1:10000 solution as a pre-filled syringe. This should be followed by a flush of sodium chloride 0.9%. If intravenous access is not available but the patient has been intubated, 2 mg can be given via the ET tube. The next set of shocks should be delivered after one minute of CPR and this should not be delayed. Only if there is time, 300 mg of amiodarone should be given intravenously, followed by a 20 ml flush of 0.9% sodium chloride. This cannot be given via the ET tube. Amiodarone works by slowing and stabilising the heart.

Three minutes later, the patient is successfully defibrillated into a sinus rhythm of a rate of 70 bpm but remains pulseless. **What drugs might be considered?**

Pulseless electrical activity is present. CPR should be commenced. A further dose of adrenaline/epinephrine is due but this should be withheld for a further minute, in case the PEA is due to myocardial stunning. In the absence of specific indications, no drugs should be given.

After a minute of CPR, the heart rate drops to 35 bpm. The team leader asks for 500 μg of atropine to be given intravenously and for the blood pressure to be checked. The cardiac arrest trolley only contains atropine in pre-filled syringes of 3 mg in 10 ml. **What volume of the pre-filled syringe should be given?**

1.67 ml should be given (1.5 ml = 0.45 mg).

Table 10.3 Drugs commonly used during resuscitation.

Drug	Indications	Dosages	Mode of action	ET	Notes
Adrenaline/epinephrine	During CPR	1 mg IV	Vasoconstricts – augments CPR	Y	Avoid administration for one minute after successful defibrillation.
	Anaphylaxis	0.5 mg IM	Vasoconstricts – increases SVR and BP		Arrhythmogenic
	Symptomatic bradycardia while awaiting transvenous pacing	2–10 µg/min	Beta-agonist – increases heart rate		
Atropine	Asystole and heart rate less than 60 in PEA	3 mg	Blocks parasympathetic activity	Y	3 mg maximum dose causes total vagal blockade
	Symptomatic bradycardia	500 mg			Repeat as required to maximum dose
Amiodarone	Refractory VF/VT	300 mg	Increases action potential	N	Give after 3 unsuccessful shocks
	Tachyarrhythmias	150 mg over 10 min or 300 mg over 1 hour			Max daily dose 1.2 g. Infusion often required
Lignocaine (lidocaine)	Refractory VF/VT	100 mg + 50 mg if necessary	Antiarrhythmic	Y	Use if amiodarone unavailable. Infusion may be necessary. Correct hypokalaemia. Caution in liver disease and the elderly
	Haemodynamically stable VT	50 mg repeated to max 200 mg			

Table 10.3 *Continued.*

Drug	Indications	Dosages	Mode of action	ET	Notes
Sodium bicarbonate	Severe acidosis Hyperkalaemia Tricyclic overdose	50 ml of 8.4%	Buffer	N	Tissue irritant. Do not give with calcium chloride
Calcium chloride	PEA associated with hyperkalaemia, hypocalcaemia, overdose of calcium channel blockers	10 ml of 10%	As a physiological buffer. Protects myocardium but won't reduce potassium levels	N	Do not give with sodium bicarbonate
Potassium chloride	Hypokalaemia	60 mmol in dilute solution	Increases serum potassium	N	Max 30 mmol per hour. Diluted in solution
Magnesium sulphate	Hypomagnesaemia Torsades de pointes	2.5 g	Increases serum magnesium	N	
Adenosine	SVT Identification tachyarrhythmia	6 mg, 12 mg	Blocks conduction through AV node temporarily	N	Unpleasant side-effects – warn patient
Naloxone	Opioid overdose	0.4–0.8 mg	Competes at opioid receptors	Y	Shorter duration of action than many opioids. May need infusion
Esmolol	SVT	40 mg	Very short-acting beta-blocker	N	Infusion may be necessary
Verapamil	SVT	5–10 mg	Calcium channel blocker	N	Avoid administering with beta-blocker

ET, endotracheal tube; SVR, systemic vascular resistance

CONCLUSION

The evidence base for the use of drugs in resuscitation is growing. Nurses and other healthcare personnel, especially those in specialist areas, are increasingly able to prevent and manage cardiac arrests, including giving drugs. Knowledge of the drug treatments available and how they are given during resuscitation will enable nurses to become more effective members of the cardiac arrest team. Table 10.3 summarises the drugs given in cardiac arrest, their actions and dosages.

REFERENCES

Adgey, A.A.J. (1998) Adrenaline/epinephrine dosage and buffers in cardiac arrest. *Heart* **80** (4), 412–14.

Bar-Joseph, G., Abramson, N.S., Jansen-McWilliams, L. *et al*. (2002) Brain resuscitation clinical trial III (BRCT III) Study Group: clinical use of sodium bicarbonate during cardiopulmonary resuscitation – is it used sensibly? *Resuscitation* **54**, 47–55.

Baskett, P. (ed.) (2000) International guidelines 2000 for CPR and ECC. A consensus on science. *Resuscitation* **46** (1–3), 1–447.

Bottiger, B.W. & Martin, E. (2001) Thrombolytic therapy during cardiopulmonary resuscitation and the role of coagulation activation after cardiac arrest. *Current Opinion in Critical Care* **7** (3), 176–83.

British National Formulary (2003) Available online at: www.bnf.org.

Department of Health (2000) *Patient Group Directions (England Only)*. Health Service Circular 2000/026. Department of Health, London.

Dorian, P., Cass, D., Schartz Cooper, B., Gelaznikas, R. & Barr, A. (2002) Amiodarone as compared with lidocaine for shock resistant ventricular fibrillation. *New England Journal of Medicine* **346**, 884–90.

EPIC Project (2001) Developing national evidence – based guidelines for preventing healthcare associated infections. Guidelines for preventing infections associated with the insertion and maintenance of central venous catheters. *Journal of Hospital Infection* **47** (suppl), S47–S67. Available online at: www.doh.gov.uk/hai/epic.doc.

Gazmuri, R.J. (1999) Buffer treatment for cardiac resuscitation: putting the cart before the horse? *Critical Care Medicine* **27** (5), 875–6.

Gonzalez, E.R., Kannewurf, B.S. & Ornato, J.P. (1998) Intravenous amiodarone for ventricular arrhythmias: overview and clinical use. *Resuscitation* **39**, 33–42.

Hinchliff, S.M., Montague, S.E. & Watson, R. (1996) *Physiology for Nursing Practice*, 2nd edn. Baillière Tindall, London.

Hinds, C.J. & Watson, D. (1996) *Intensive Care: A Concise Textbook*. W.B. Saunders, London.

Hopkins, S.J. (1999) *Drugs and Pharmacology for Nurses*, 13th edn. Churchill Livingstone, Edinburgh.

Johnstone, S.L., Unsworth, J. & Gompels, M.M. (2003) Adrenaline/epinephrine given outside the context of life threatening allergic reactions. *British Medical Journal* **326**, 589–90.

Jowett, N.I., Turner, A.M., Hawkings, D. & Denham, N. (2001) Emergency drug availability for the cardiac arrest team: a national audit. *Resuscitation* **4**, 179–81.

Krismer, A.C., Wenzel, V., Mayr, V.D. *et al.* (2001) Arginine vasopressin during cardiopulmonary resuscitation and vasodilatory shock: current experience and future prospects. *Current Opinion in Critical Care* **7**, 157–69.

Kudenchuk, P.J., Cobb, L.A., Copass, M.K. *et al.* (1999) Amiodarone for resuscitation after out of hospital cardiac arrest due to ventricular fibrillation. *New England Journal of Medicine* **341**, 871–8.

Lamb, J.F., Ingram, C.G., Johnston, I.A. & Pitman, R.M. (1991) *Essentials of Physiology*, 3rd edn. Blackwell Scientific Publications, London.

Lockey, A.S. & Nolan, J.P. (2001) Cardiopulmonary resuscitation in adults: revised guidelines are more evidence based. *British Medical Journal* **323**, 819–20.

Mader, T.J., Bertloet, B., Ornato, J.P. & Gutterman, J.M. (2000) Aminophylline in the treatment of atropine resistant bradyasystole. *Resuscitation* **47**, 105–12.

Madrid, P. & Sendlebach, S. (2001) Heart-smarter drugs for resuscitation: an update on ACLS algorithms – drug changes introduced at the historic 2000 conference. *American Journal of Nursing* **101** (5), S42–S44.

Manisterski, Y., Vaknin, Z., Ben-Abraham, R. *et al.* (2002) Endotracheal epinephrine: a call for larger doses. *Anesthesia and Analgesia* **95** (4), 1037–41.

NHSE North West (2003) *Patient Group Directions (PGDs) – Approved Group Protocols*. Available online at: www.groupprotocols.org.uk.

Niemann, J.T. & Stratton, S.J. (2000) Endotracheal versus intravenous epinephrine and atropine in out of hospital 'primary' and postcountershock asystole. *Critical Care Medicine* **28** (6), 1815–19.

Niemann, J.T., Stratton, S.J., Cruz, B. & Lewis, R.J. (2002) Endotracheal drug administration during out of hospital resuscitation: where are the survivors? *Resuscitation* **53**, 153–7.

Nursing and Midwifery Council (2002) *Guidelines for the Administration of Medicines*. Nursing and Midwifery Council, London.

Nolan, J.P., de Latorre, F.J., Steen, P.A., Chamberlain, D.A. & Bossaert, L.L. (2002) Advanced life support drugs: do they really work? *Current Opinion in Critical Care* **8**, 212–18.

Polderman, K.H. & Girbes, A.R.J. (2002) Central venous catheter use. Part 1: mechanical complications. *Intensive Care Medicine* **28**, 1–17.

Prengel, A.W., Rembecki, M., Wenzel, V. & Steinbach, G. (2001) A comparison of the endotracheal tube and the laryngeal mask airway as a route for endobronchial lidocaine administration. *Anesthesia and Analgesia* **92** (6), 1505–9.

Prosser, S., Worster, B., MacGregor, J., Dewar, K., Runyard, P. & Fegan, J. (2000) *Applied Pharmacology: An Introduction to Pathophysiology and Drug Management for Nurses and Healthcare Professionals.* Mosby, Edinburgh.

Resuscitation Council UK (2000) *Advanced Life Support Course Provider Manual*, 4th edn. Resuscitation Council UK, London.

Taylor, S.E. (2002) Amiodarone: an emergency medicine perspective. *Emergency Medicine* **14**, 422–9.

Woodrow, P. (2002) Central venous catheters and central venous pressure. *Nursing Standard* **16** (26), 45–52, 54.

11 | Management of Potentially Reversible Causes of Cardiac Arrest

INTRODUCTION

When a patient collapses suddenly and presents in cardiac arrest, it is vital to institute appropriate resuscitation measures. In addition, steps must be taken to identify the underlying cause, as this will enable the resuscitation ream to implement strategies to reverse or correct the causative factors. The causes of cardiac arrest in the adult patient are attributable to airway obstruction, respiratory inadequacy and cardiac abnormalities (Resuscitation Council UK 2000a), with many factors ultimately contributing to the subsequent cardiopulmonary arrest of the patient. Some, such as the obstruction of the patient's airway by the tongue falling back against the posterior pharyngeal wall, are easily remedied if the cause of the problem is identified quickly by accurate and timely assessment.

AIMS

This chapter explores the various causes for a cardiac arrest and describes the individual measures to reverse or correct the underlying problems.

LEARNING OUTCOMES

At the end of the chapter the reader should be able to:

❏ list the *reversible causes* of cardiac arrest;
❏ describe how to *recognise and respond* to key causes of reversible cardiac arrest;
❏ demonstrate understanding of the *importance* of recognising and responding to the underlying cause of cardiac arrest;
❏ demonstrate understanding of the *non-reversible causes* of cardiac arrest;

❏ describe the factors that can influence a positive outcome in a cardiac arrest situation for the patient.

CAUSES OF CARDIAC ARREST

Cardiorespiratory arrest may occur because of a primary airway, breathing or circulation problem (Resuscitation Council UK 2000a). However, it is important to remember that many life-threatening diseases can cause secondary respiratory or cardiac problems, which may ultimately result in the patient suffering a respiratory and/or cardiopulmonary arrest (see Table 11.1).

Respiratory inadequacy may be due to disorders of the respiratory system such as asthma or pulmonary oedema. A decrease in the patient's respiratory drive may be due to central nervous system depression or decreased respiratory effort because of exhaustion or drugs depressing the patient's respiratory drive. In turn, the resulting hypoxia may have a direct effect on the heart by causing a bradycardia, which causes inadequate perfusion of the brain or heart and leads to cardiac arrest (Resuscitation Council UK 2000a). Cardiac abnormalities may be a primary or contributory cause of the cardiac arrest (see Table 11.2).

Table 11.1 Causes of airway obstruction.

Blood
Vomit
Foreign body, e.g. food or a broken tooth
Direct trauma to the face
Decreased level of consciousness
Epiglottitis
Swelling to the pharynx, e.g. caused by infection
Laryngospasm
Bronchospasm
Cardiomyopathy

Table 11.2 Causes of primary cardiac arrest.

Ischaemia
Myocardial infarction
Hypertensive heart disease
Valve disease
Drugs (e.g. antiarrhythmic drugs, tricyclic antidepressants, digoxin)
Acidosis
Abnormal electrolyte concentration
Hypothermia
Electrocution (which can cause paralysis of the respiratory muscles or send the
    patient into VF or asystole)
Cardiac failure
Cardiac tamponade
Cardiac rupture
Myocarditis

A secondary cardiac abnormality is one where the heart is affected by a problem originating elsewhere (Resuscitation Council UK 2000a). Thus cardiac arrest may occur following:

- asphyxia from airway obstruction or apnoea
- tension pneumothorax
- hypovolaemia
- hypothermia
- severe septic shock.

The treatment of any potentially reversible cause of a cardiac arrest is of paramount importance irrespective of the underlying rhythm. The most recent resuscitation guidelines (Resuscitation Council UK 2000b) highlight the importance of considering reversible causes in *all* cardiac arrest rhythms.

The reversible causes of cardiac arrest can be most easily remembered as 'the four Hs and four Ts', as shown in Table 11.3.

An important part of the process of resuscitation is the gathering of clues to piece together as much history as possible in order to elicit the cause or causes of the cardiac arrest. Thus the team leader directing the resuscitation process may try to elicit further information about the events leading up to the point of cardiac arrest in the patient.

Table 11.3 Reversible causes of cardiac arrest, the four Hs and four Ts.

Hypoxia
Hypovolaemia
Hyperkalaemia/hypokalaemia (and other metabolic disorders)
Hypothermia
Tension pneumothorax
Tamponade
Thromboembolic
Toxic/therapeutic disturbances

- Was there a history of trauma prior to the event?
- Does the patient suffer from any underlying disease processes, which may have been a contributory factor to their collapsed state?
- Does the patient take any prescribed (or non-prescribed) medication?
- Have environmental factors been a contributory factor to the collapse? Where was the patient found? When had they last been seen conscious by a witness?

MANAGING THE REVERSIBLE CAUSES OF CARDIAC ARREST

Hypoxia

Recognition
All patients who experience a cardiopulmonary arrest will have suffered some degree of hypoxia. Understanding the events leading up to the time of arrest will enable the team to discover whether it was the result of a primary cardiac event, such as a myocardial infarction, or whether it occurred at the end of a long period of physiological compensation. For example, the patient who experienced respiratory failure as a result of a severe exacerbation of asthma will present with the following signs and symptoms.

- Tachypnoea (respiratory rate of greater than 30 breaths per minute or a respiratory rate of 10 breaths or less a minute).
- Exhaustion.

- Tachycardia or bradycardia.
- Hypotension.
- Reduced conscious level.
- Falling PaO_2, despite oxygen therapy.
- Rising $PaCO_2$, despite therapy (Advanced Life Support Group 2001).

Response
In order to prevent further hypoxia and to try to reverse the damaging effects of hypoxia on the myocardium, the patient needs to be oxygenated as effectively as possible. This may be achieved by ventilating the patient. This initially might involve a bag-valve-mask connected to high-flow oxygen (12–15 litres per minute) and ensuring adequate rise and fall of the chest.

- The gold standard is to secure the patient's airway with an endotracheal (ET) tube. However, expertise in this area is required and the hypoxia may be compounded while the ET tube is being passed. An alternative which may be considered in this situation is the insertion of a laryngeal mask airway (LMA).
- If the patient is intubated it is essential that regular checks are carried out during the resuscitation to ensure the ET tube does not become misplaced into a bronchus or oesophagus.
- Misplacement of the ET tube will compound the hypoxia suffered by the patient.

Hypovolaemia

Recognition
The history precipitating the cardiac arrest may suggest severe volume loss, such as trauma due to rupture of the liver or spleen, gastrointestinal bleeding or rupture of an aortic aneurysm. The signs and symptoms of hypovolaemia are illustrated in Table 11.4.

Response
Replacement of intravascular volume is of paramount importance while advanced life support continues.

Table 11.4 Signs and symptoms of hypovolaemia.

Tachycardia (rate >100 beats per minute)
Hypotension
Sweating
Pallor
Agitation
Thready or unpalpable distal pulses
Prolonged capillary refill time (>2 seconds)

- For severe cases, a large-bore cannula should be placed into each antecubital fossa of the patient.
- The cannulae should be at least 16 G or 14 G in order to allow large amounts of fluid to be administered quickly.
- An alternative position for easy access is the external jugular vein of the patient. Two litres of crystalloid or colloid can then be administered as quickly as possible.
- There has been much controversy about the choice of fluid to be used in an emergency situation (Alderson *et al.* 2003). Saline 0.9%, Hartmann's solution or a colloid such as Gelofusin or Haemacel are all acceptable.
- The aim is to replace approximately 40% of the patient's circulating volume as quickly as possible.
- In high-dependency areas such as the emergency department, intensive care unit and theatres, infusion pumps may be available that can deliver 2 litres of warmed fluid to the patient in less than five minutes.
- Having administered the fluid, it is important to remember to reassess the effect at appropriate intervals in the algorithm. This is especially important if the patient is in pulseless electrical activity (PEA), as a palpable pulse may then be felt after this intervention.
- If the underlying cause of the cardiac arrest was haemorrhage, urgent surgery may be required if the resuscitation is successful in order to stop the haemorrhage.

Table 11.5 Normal serum electrolyte levels.

Electrolyte	Normal range
Potassium	3.5–5.0 mmol/l
Magnesium	>0.7 mmol/l
Calcium	0.85–1.4 mmol/l (with albumin corrected)

Hyperkalaemia, hypocalcaemia and metabolic disorders

Recognition

The cause of a cardiac arrest may be a metabolic disorder, often an electrolyte imbalance. The clinical history may alert the team to the underlying problem. Suspicion of the diagnosis may be confirmed through the measurement of arterial blood gases but serum electrolytes will provide more objective data (see Table 11.5). The ECG can also be used as an adjunct to the diagnosis.

- For example, if a patient suffered from renal failure this may lead to suspicions of a raised potassium level. A 12-lead ECG taken previously may be helpful. Peaked T waves, broad QRS complexes and conduction defects are also indicative of a high potassium level (Connaughton 2001), whereas ECG changes in hypokalaemia may include ST depression, flattening of the T wave and a prominent U wave (Whiteley *et al*. 1998).

- From the arterial blood sample, it is possible to determine the severity of acidosis following a cardiac arrest and also the measurement of key electrolytes, including potassium levels.

- If the patient presents having taken an overdose of calcium channel blockers, this may lead the team to think of hypocalcaemia being the cause of the cardiac arrest and this may be reversed by giving calcium chloride.

- In hypocalcaemia, signs and symptoms a patient may exhibit prior to cardiac arrest include convulsions, depressed cardiac function, muscle weakness, paraesthesia, tetany and ECG changes such as a prolonged QT interval (Womack 2002).

Response
- In all cases continuous ECG monitoring should be instigated along with frequent observations and reassessment of the patient. A baseline blood test for urea and electrolyte measurement should be taken and this will be repeated at regular intervals.
- In hyperkalaemia, calcium chloride 10 ml of 10% should be administered intravenously in order to lower the extracellular potassium quickly and prevent any life-threatening arrhythmia.
- In hypokalaemia, potassium chloride can be given as prescribed, diluted in saline via a central line.
- In hypocalcaemia, 10 ml of 10% calcium chloride is given by slow bolus (Whiteley *et al.* 1998).

Magnesium abnormalities are frequently associated with other electrolyte abnormalities such as hypocalcaemia. Calcium and magnesium excretion are interdependent. Hypomagnesaemia can also cause refractory ventricular fibrillation and if suspected, should be treated by giving intravenous magnesium to correct the electrolyte imbalance. Calcium chloride is also indicated if hypermagnesaemia is suspected (Womack 2002).

Hypothermia

Recognition
Hypothermia is defined as a core temperature less than 35°C (Steedman 1994).

Mild to moderate hypothermia is defined as a core temperature of 30–32°C and severe hypothermia as a core temperature of below 30°C (Guly & Richardson 1996).

- If there is rapid cooling prior to the development of hypoxia, decreased oxygen consumption and metabolism may precede the cardiac arrest and reduce organ ischaemia (Larach 1995). Therefore becoming cold very quickly can exert a protective effect on the brain and other vital organs during cardiac arrest (Larach 1995).

- Using a tympanic thermometer will give a fast reading to confirm the diagnosis. Oesophageal temperature monitoring may be used in a critical care area.

It is imperative to record the patient's temperature as soon as possible as it will directly affect the management of the cardiac arrest. If the first three shocks in pulseless ventricular tachycardia or ventricular fibrillation (VF/VT) are unsuccessful, then further attempts at defibrillation should be deferred until the core temperature is greater than 30°C (Resuscitation Council UK 2000a), as they are very unlikely to be successful and will simply cause further damage to the myocardium.

In PEA the ECG may show evidence of J waves. These are seen at the junction of the QRS complex and ST segments. They are thought to be due to hypothermia-induced ion fluxes causing delayed left ventricular depolarisation or early repolarisation (Steedman 1994).

Drugs should also be withheld until the core temperature is above 30°C, as administration will simply lead to pooling of the drugs in the peripheral circulation without any direct action on the heart.

Response

Once the diagnosis is established, passive rewarming methods such as using warm blankets will be ineffective if the patient has lost their cardiac output (Larach 1995). Active and rapid rewarming is essential in order to reverse the cause of the cardiac arrest (Carson 1999). Active rewarming includes:

- the administration of warmed (42–46°C) and humidified oxygen;
- administering warmed (40–43°C) intravenous fluids;
- catheterising the patient and carrying out a bladder washout with warmed fluids;
- peritoneal lavage with warmed fluid (which must be potassium free);
- the gold standard is extracorporeal blood warming (by-pass) but only a small percentage of hospitals can offer this treatment. It would only be available in centres where cardiac

by-pass operations or haemodialysis are offered (Wollenek *et al*. 2002).

It is important to remember that during a prolonged arrest, a patient who was normothermic may become hypothermic (Resuscitation Council UK 2000a).

Tension pneumothorax

Recognition

A tension pneumothorax develops when air enters the pleural space as a result of a laceration to the lung, bronchus or chest wall. The airflow is unidirectional, which means that air flows into the pleural space on inspiration but cannot escape during expiration due to the effective formation of a one-way valve. This causes a progressive accumulation of air in the pleura; the lung will collapse and the pressure will continue to build up, pushing the mediastinum to the opposite side. This in turn reduces venous return, resulting in a low or ineffective cardiac output (Greaves *et al*. 2001).

Tension pnuemothorax is a clinical diagnosis. There is no time to confirm the presence of a tension pneumothorax through a chest X-ray. The signs which indicate a tension pneumothorax is present are:

- decreased or absent air entry in the affected side of the chest;
- hyper-resonance on percussion of the affected side of the chest;
- tracheal deviation (away from the affected side);
- distended neck veins (although this is absent in the hypovolaemic patient).

A tension pneumothorax may be suspected in a patient who has suffered chest trauma or asthma or has recently had a central line inserted.

Response

A needle thoracocentesis or needle decompression should be carried out by the medical team. A large-bore cannula is inserted into the second intercostal space in the mid-clavicular line on the affected side of the chest. Later on, a chest drain will need to be inserted (see Figure 11.1).

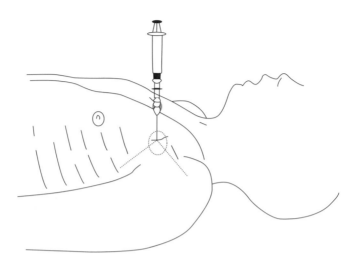

Fig. 11.1 Landmarks for insertion of cannula.

Cardiac tamponade

Recognition

In cardiac tamponade, blood fills the pericardial space which in turn raises intrapericardial pressure, compressing the heart and preventing it from expanding. As a result there is reduced cardiac output (Nolan & Gwinnutt 1998).

Clinical features of cardiac tamponade include:

- raised jugular venous pressure (JVP);
- hypotension;
- tachycardia;
- muffled heart sounds;
- pulsus paradoxus.

The classic clinical features of distended neck veins, hypotension and muffled heart sounds are absent in cardiac arrest. The preceding history and an account of the mechanism of injury are therefore important. Suspicion should be aroused if the patient has suffered any trauma to the thorax and complains of chest pain.

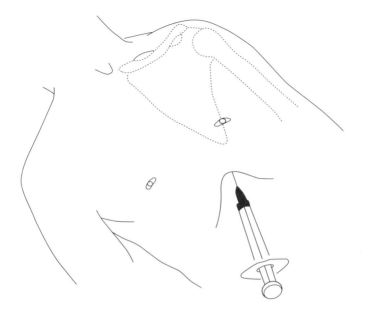

Fig. 11.2 Pericardiocentesis.

Response
In order to treat this cause of cardiac arrest, a needle pericardiocentesis must be performed as an emergency procedure. An attempt is made to aspirate blood from the pericardial sac in order to enable the heart to fill again and produce a palpable cardiac output (see Figure 11.2). The patient would then need to undergo emergency cardiac surgery.

Thromboembolic or mechanical obstruction

Recognition
The most common cause of thromboembolic or mechanical obstruction causing the patient to lose their cardiac output is a massive pulmonary embolus. It has been suggested that an emergency pulmonary embolectomy (removal of the clot) can

be life saving (Resuscitation Council UK 2000a). In practice, this is not a procedure commonly carried out. There does appear to be a growing body of evidence that thrombolysis (giving clot-busting drugs) during the resuscitation may be helpful (Caldicott *et al.* 2002).

Signs of a pulmonary embolus before a patient loses cardiac output include:

- chest pain
- shortness of breath
- cyanosis
- haemoptysis.

Toxic/therapeutic disturbances

Recognition
Poisoning is a leading cause of cardiac arrest in younger adults (Resuscitation Council UK 2000a). The drugs may have a negatively inotropic effect on the heart. Alternatively, cardiac arrest may be a secondary endpoint caused by respiratory failure or central nervous system depression (Nelson & Hoffman 1996).

There may be a definitive history of accidental or deliberate ingestion of therapeutic or toxic substances such as an overdose of tablets or exposure to carbon monoxide. However, even if there is no specific evidence of poisoning, it should be considered as the cause of cardiac arrest in every collapsed patient. The hospital team should ensure that they are not put at risk if chemical or radiation exposure from the patient is a possibility.

Response
- The emphasis is on intensive supportive therapy, with correction of hypoxia, acidosis and electrolyte disorders (Resuscitation Council UK 2000a).
- If the ingested drug can be identified then the National Poison Centre can be consulted to see if a specific antidote is indicated (see Table 11.6). However, perhaps surprisingly, there are few specific antidotes available.

- An important factor to be taken into consideration is the fact that this group of patients is usually younger and therefore less likely to suffer from concurrent heart disease. The resuscitation may be prolonged as the poison may be metabolised or excreted during advanced life support (Resuscitation Council UK 2000a).

Non-reversible causes of cardiac arrest

There are occasions when despite the best efforts of the resuscitation team, a positive outcome for the patient is not possible due to the primary cause of the cardiopulmonary arrest. Such causes may be divided into cardiac and non-cardiac pathology.

Cardiac causes

- Mitral valve prolapse.
- Hypertrophic myopathy.
- Massive myocardial infarction affecting a critical mass of myocardium.
- Continuous asystole despite advanced life support measures for more than 20 minutes in a normothermic patient.
- Patients who have received no resuscitation for at least 15 minutes after collapse.

Non-cardiac causes

- Massive trauma, such as massive cranial and cerebral destruction (Hillman 2003).
- Submersion in water for more than three hours in adults (Resuscitation Council UK 2000a).

Table 11.6 Specific antidotes used to treat overdose.

Drug/poison	Specific antidote
Tricyclic antidepressants	Sodium bicarbonate if ECG changes occur
Opioids	Naloxone
Cocaine toxicity	Benzodiazepines
Beta-blockers	Glucagon
Organophosphates (weed killer)	Atropine

(Resuscitation Council (UK) 2000a)

REVIEW OF LEARNING

❏ It is essential that effective basic life support and advanced life support are ongoing throughout a resuscitation.

❏ In order to aid a positive outcome, it is important to consider any or all of the potential reversible causes of cardiac arrest.

❏ These can be remembered as the 'four Hs and four Ts'.

❏ Even when every reversible cause is sought and treated, there may be occasions when despite the best efforts of the resuscitation team, the outcome for the patient is unsuccessful. This can particularly be the case when the cardiac arrest was caused by a catastrophic, irrecoverable event.

Case study

Mr Brown was admitted to the ward from the emergency department two hours ago. He has suffered from an exacerbation of asthma and was initially stabilised with continuous nebulised salbutamol. He was maintaining his oxygen saturations at 90–92% on 15 litres of oxygen via a non-rebreathing mask. You go to administer a nebuliser and find him unresponsive and pulseless. **What are your actions?**

On assessment of airway, breathing and circulation, the patient is found to be apnoeic and pulseless. The cardiac arrest team is called and basic life support is commenced. The monitor is connected and the rhythm is found to be PEA at a rate of 40. **What should be the actions of the team now?**

The patient has been intubated and has received 1 mg adrenaline and 3 mg atropine. Cardiac compressions and ventilation are now being carried out continuously. (One potentially reversible cause of cardiac arrest has been addressed – hypoxia.)

Can you think of any other reversible causes of the cardiac arrest in this situation?

On reassessment, a thready pulse is felt. The patient is stabilised and moved to the intensive care unit for continuing care.

CONCLUSION

The seriously ill patient presents many challenges and being able to assess the signs of an impending cardiac arrest demands great skill. However, if preventive measures fail and the patient suffers a cardiac arrest, basic life support must be instituted as quickly as possible, followed by advanced life support. When it is established that the cause for collapse is not cardiac, but originating elsewhere, the additional underlying causes of the arrest must then be considered and addressed. Systematic analysis of the reversible causes of a cardiac arrest will enable rescuers to recognise the precipitating factors, intervene appropriately and influence survival outcomes.

REFERENCES

Advanced Life Support Group (2001) *Acute Medical Emergencies.* BMJ Books, London.

Alderson, P., Schierhout, G., Roberts, I. & Bunn, F. (2003) Colloids versus crystalloids for fluid resuscitation in critically ill patients (Cochrane Review). In: *The Cochrane Library*, Issue 2, Oxford.

Caldicott, D., Parasivam, S., Harding, J., Edwards, N. & Bochner, F. (2002) Tenectplase for massive pulmonary embolus. *Resuscitation* **33**, 211–13.

Carson, B. (1999) Successful resuscitation of a 44-year-old man with hypothermia. *Journal of Emergency Nursing* **25**, 356 60.

Connaughton, M. (2001) *Evidence-Based Coronary Care.* Churchill Livingstone, London.

Greaves, I., Porter, K. & Ryan, J. (2001) *Trauma Care Manual.* Arnold, London.

Guly, U. & Richardson, D. (1996) *Acute Medical Emergencies.* Oxford University Press, Oxford.

Hillman, H. (2003) The physiology of sudden violent death. *Resuscitation* **56**, 129–33.

Larach, M. (1995) Accidental hypothermia. *Lancet* **345**, 493–8.

Nelson, L. & Hoffman, R. (1996) *Toxicologic sudden death.* In: Paradis, N., Halperin, H. & Nowak, R. (eds) *Cardiac Arrest: the Science and Practice of Resuscitation Medicine.* Williams and Wilkins, London.

Nolan, J.P. & Gwinnutt, C. (1998) 1998 European guidelines on resuscitation. *British Medical Journal* **316**, 1844–5.

Resuscitation Council UK (2000a) *Advanced Life Support Provider Manual*, 4th edn. Resuscitation Council UK, London.

Resuscitation Council UK (2000b) *Resuscitation Guidelines 2000.* Resuscitation Council UK, London.

Steedman, D. (1994) *Environmental Medical Emergencies.* Oxford University Press, Oxford.

Whiteley, S., Bodeham, A. & Bellamy, M. (1998) *Intensive Care.* Churchill Livingstone, London.

Wollenek, G., Honarwar, N., Golej, J. & Marx, M. (2002) Cold water submersion and cardiac arrest in treatment of serve hypothermia with cardiopulmonary bypass. *Resuscitation* **52**, 255–63.

Womack, K. (2002) Fluids and electrolytes. In: Newberry L. (ed.) *Sheehy's Emergency Nursing, Principles and Practice.* Mosby, St Louis.

Post-Resuscitation Care

12

INTRODUCTION

For every 100 inpatient cardiac arrests, approximately 45 will be successfully resuscitated and achieve return of spontaneous circulation (ROSC) but only around 17 are likely to survive to discharge from hospital (Gwinnutt *et al*. 2000).

The degree of existing acute and chronic disease and also the damage caused by the arrest will both influence short- and long-term survival; however, early recognition of problems coupled with a rapid response will increase the likelihood of a successful outcome (Langhelle *et al*. 2003). Post-resuscitation care should be thought of as continued resuscitation care and aims to stabilise cardiac performance, optimise tissue perfusion to the vital organs and minimise brain damage.

AIMS

This chapter describes the key principles of post-resuscitation care and approaches for improving long-term survival.

LEARNING OUTCOMES

At the end of the chapter the reader should be able to:

❏ understand the importance of a *continued structured approach* to care of the patient in the post-resuscitation phase;
❏ demonstrate knowledge of the *principles of monitoring*;
❏ describe common methods of *monitoring the patient*;
❏ demonstrate awareness of *common post-resuscitation investigations*;
❏ describe priorities associated with *safe patient transfer*;
❏ discuss important issues relating to *care of relatives and staff* following resuscitation.

POST-RESUSCITATION TREATMENT

How unstable is the post-resuscitation patient?

The casualty sustaining a witnessed ventricular fibrillation (VF) arrest who receives a precordial thump to restore a normal rhythm may have had an arrest lasting less than 30 seconds and may not suffer any further complications. In contrast, the hospitalised patient with an infective exacerbation of chronic obstructive pulmonary disease who has a cardiac arrest will need lengthy advanced life support and require complex and aggressive management in the post-resuscitation phase. Factors affecting post-arrest physiological patient stability and outcomes of resuscitation are detailed in Chapter 9, Table 9.1.

Post-resuscitation treatment aims to:

- optimise tissue perfusion, particularly of the heart and brain;
- identify the cause of arrest;
- prevent further arrest;
- enable safe transfer of patient to the most appropriate area.

Post-resuscitation management

Oxygen delivery to the tissues depends on proper management of airway, breathing and circulation. A structured assessment using the 'A–E' model (see Chapter 2) followed by a systematic approach to monitoring may allow recognition and response to any further cardiac arrests in this extremely vulnerable group.

MONITORING

There are some basic rules of monitoring, as seen in Table 12.1.

Airway/breathing

Observing the patient's level of consciousness, chest movement, respiratory rate and noise of breathing will all yield important information. This will be of even greater significance in association with recordings of, for example, blood pressure and heart rate.

Following a cardiac arrest, patients can be sufficiently alert to adequately maintain their own airway. Alternatively some may have been intubated during resuscitation and will require the endotracheal tube to remain in place for a short period during the post-resuscitation phase.

Assisted ventilation may be required in the period after the arrest for the following reasons:

- apnoea;
- spontaneous breathing inadequate, breaths are too slow or shallow;
- oxygen and carbon dioxide levels require alteration and optimisation;
- patient unable to maintain required work of breathing;
- stabilise the patient's cardiopulmonary status.

The process of respiration enables oxygen uptake and the removal of carbon dioxide. It is obviously essential to deliver adequate levels of oxygen in order to prevent tissue hypoxia, which can increase the risk of further arrest and also deprive the brain of vital oxygen supplies.

In certain circumstances excessive assisted ventilation or hyperventilation by the patient can lead to a fall in carbon dioxide (CO_2) levels (hypocarbia). This can lead to a reduction in blood flow to the brain (Resuscitation Council UK 2000).

Table 12.1 Basic rules of monitoring.

Machines are fallible; always check the patient	• Poor contact of monitoring electrodes may cause a picture of asystole to appear on the monitor
Using machines to monitor patients does not replace basic clinical skills and close observation	• Changes in patient's mental status, skin colour and skin temperature will not be detected by cardiac monitoring and recording blood pressure
The readings and their significance must be understood by the nurse recording them	• Those caring for patients on cardiac monitors must have skills to recognise changes in rhythm and respond appropriately
Trends are more important than one-off measurement in determining whether patient is improving or deteriorating	• A heart rate of 60 beats per minute is likely to be entirely normal; however, it would be hugely significant if it had been 120 one hour earlier

Oxygen saturation

Arterial oxygen saturation (SaO_2) describes the percentage of haemoglobin that is saturated with oxygen and is a useful measure of oxygen delivery. An SaO_2 of 97% indicates 97% of the total haemoglobin in the blood contains molecules of oxygen (Moore 2004). However, the patient with a low haemoglobin may have a very high oxygen saturation, even though the oxygen-carrying capacity of the blood is greatly reduced. Oxygen saturation monitors do not measure CO_2 levels nor do they offer any guidance on respiratory performance. The saturation sensor is usually placed on an area that is well perfused, such as the tip of the finger or ear lobe. If perfusion to that extremity is reduced the probe will not pick up a trace and will alarm for this reason and not because the saturation has necessarily dropped (Howell 2002). Other factors that can affect the trace include:

- patient movement, restlessness;
- dark skin pigmentation, jaundice and high serum bilirubin levels;
- blood, dirt or (blue or black) nail polish between sensor and finger;
- dysrhythmias;
- anaemia or abnormal haemoglobin.

Circulation

Inadequate circulation can be the cause or the consequence of cardiac arrest. It is essential to regularly assess blood pressure, pulse and respiration in order to recognise cardiac dysfunction and rhythm instability, which may follow an arrest and will require support until adequate perfusion has been re-established. It is worth noting that a rising respiratory rate is one of the earliest signs of circulatory failure.

Cardiac monitoring

Chapter 8 explained that the electrocardiogram (ECG) trace may be entirely normal in the presence of a cardiac arrest. This reinforces the point that the patient should be the focus of attention, not the monitor. Alterations in the rate and rhythm may be of cardiac origin or may reflect dysfunction in other systems, for example in the lungs or in electrolytes. Changes in the cardiac rhythm may be very dramatic and sudden, such as the onset of ventricular fibrillation (VF), or may be more subtle, such as a gradual rise in heart rate due to bleeding. The monitor will usefully detect changes, as seen in Table 12.2.

Central venous pressure monitoring

Central venous pressure (CVP) is the pressure in the central veins (caused by blood volume) as it enters the right atrium of the heart. It provides a measure of the circulating volume in the body. Measurement of the CVP assists the nurse in optimising pressures in the right and left sides of the heart. In right heart failure fluids may be needed to stretch the right ventricle to make the heart work more efficiently. Alternatively, in left heart failure diuretics and nitrates may be required to reduce the workload of the left ventricle, resulting in a predicted fall in CVP.

Table 12.2 Monitoring ECG changes.

Rhythm disturbance	Examples of possible cause
Irregular heart rhythm	• Hypoxia • Myocardial ischaemia • Heart block • Atrial fibrillation (AF) • Malfunctioning artificial pacemaker
Widening QRS complexes	• Rhythm originating in the ventricles • Bundle branch block • Electrolyte imbalance • Poisoning • Hypothermia
Lengthening PR interval	• Deterioration of AV node function
P waves independent from QRS complexes	• Absence of conduction across AV node (complete heart block)

It is essential that all CVP measurements be taken from the same place, either the sternal angle or from the mid-axillae, where the fourth intercostal space and mid-axillary line intersect (Woodrow 2004). However, changes in patient position, hyperinflation of the lungs, over-hydration and dehydration may also alter CVP readings.

Disability

The patient's neurological function should be assessed immediately after the return of spontaneous circulation. This should include:

- Glasgow Coma Score (see Chapter 14, Table 14.4);
- blood glucose.

Glasgow Coma Scale

Used to assess and identify trends in neurological function based on specific body responses. Patients who are fully alert score 15 and those in a coma score 3.

Exposure

Exposure and head-to-toe examination will be used to assess other aspects of the patient's existing pathology that may have caused or contributed to the cardiac arrest. Checking wounds, drains and the skin for signs of infection or dehydration may be of great significance.

Specialised monitoring

The following systems of monitoring are specialised and are most commonly seen in critical care areas such as intensive therapy units (ITU).

Capnography

When a patient has been intubated a capnograph will measure the level of carbon dioxide in the exhaled air from the patient's lungs. Carbon dioxide is not produced by the stomach so the presence of CO_2 will assist in confirming that the ET tube is in the trachea and not the oesophagus. Continuous capnography is not only a constant confirmation that the ET tube is in the correct place, for example during patient transfer, but will also reflect heart–lung function because if tissues are not effectively perfused only small amounts of CO_2 will be excreted. Thus capnography reflects the adequacy of circulation (Schnell & Puntillo 2001).

Arterial pressure monitoring

This is a continuous and extremely accurate means of monitoring the systolic and diastolic blood pressure. It is used in critical care settings to assess the patient's response to the therapies they are given in the immediate post-resuscitation phase.

The pressures are displayed as continuous traces on a monitor.

INVESTIGATIONS

The same rules apply to investigations as to monitoring. There is no value to a 12-lead ECG or chest X-ray unless someone with experience is available to interpret them.

Twelve-lead ECG

Electrocardiogram monitoring provides continuous information about the heart's electrical activity (see Chapter 8), whereas the benefit of a 12-lead ECG is that it produces 12 'views' of the heart and will record the electrical activity from three dimensions. Additionally, not all heart-related problems can be displayed via a cardiac monitor so a 12-lead ECG is necessary to reveal these. For example, bundle branch blocks or myocardial ischaemia are easier to diagnose with a 12-lead ECG.

The 12-lead ECG can assist in investigating many clinical conditions, including:

- finer points of unstable rhythms and the conduction system;
- acute coronary syndromes (ACS);
- evidence of previous myocardial infarction;
- structural heart damage;
- other conditions such as pulmonary embolus, chronic obstructive pulmonary disease, digoxin toxicity, electrolyte disorders.

Table 12.3 Commonly requested post-resuscitation blood tests.

Test	Reasons for test include
Urea and creatinine	• Assist assessment of renal function • Extent of dehydration
Blood chemistry	• Identify abnormalities in potassium, sodium, calcium, etc.
Cardiac enzymes	• Identifying extent of cardiac muscle damage • Determining risk of ischaemic damage
Serum glucose	• Important to maintain at normal levels
Full blood count	• Identify risk or extent of bleeding

Blood tests

A great many tests may be conducted on blood taken from the post-arrest patient (see Table 12.3).

Arterial blood gases (ABG)

All the tests listed in Table 12.3 are usually measured from a blood sample from a vein (venous). By definition, an arterial blood sample is taken from an artery. Blood pressure in the arteries is much higher than in the veins so bleeding occurs from the puncture site more profusely and for much longer and so firm pressure for an extended time is required after the sample is taken.

The ABG is used to:

• evaluate derangements of acid–base balance;
• establish levels of blood oxygenation and CO_2 elimination;
• assess whether the underlying problem is respiratory or metabolic.

Normal metabolism creates a slight excess of acidic compounds, which are normally excreted by the kidneys and also the process of respiration. Cells of the body require a degree of acidosis/alkalosis that is normal or close to normal (Driscoll *et al.* 1997).

During a cardiac arrest an acidaemia is likely to develop due to:

- build-up of lactic acid as the tissues are starved of oxygen (metabolic);
- build-up of CO_2 as it cannot be removed by the lungs (respiratory).

The post-arrest patient is highly likely to be suffering from an acidaemia that is both metabolic and respiratory in origin.

Chest X-ray
In this situation the chest X-ray is used to examine the cause for concern prior to the arrest or any potential damage caused during the resuscitation (see Table 12.4).

TRANSFER
It is almost certain that the patient who has sustained a cardiac arrest will need to be transferred following the event. Even if the arrest occurred in an environment such as the intensive care unit, the patient may require transfer to theatre and/or X-ray for diagnostic imaging. Whatever the length of the journey to be travelled, the same principles still apply.

Stabilisation prior to departure
Prior to departure, the team leader must ensure that the patient's airway, breathing and circulation have been stabilised. Experienced personnel must be available to ensure that the patient transfer is well co-ordinated and managed.

Table 12.4 Chest X-ray assessment.

Lungs	• Pneumothorax or haemothorax • Pulmonary oedema • Pleural effusion
Heart	• Size and shape will assist diagnosis of heart failure
Bones	• Rib fractures
Tubes and lines inserted during resuscitation	• ET tube • Central venous line • Nasogastric tube • Temporary pacing wire

Patient transfer is a dangerous time for a number of reasons:

- less support available from experienced colleagues;
- poor working environment, space and light;
- movement may displace tubes and lines;
- often less equipment, only limited amount can be carried;
- if something breaks or oxygen runs out, difficult to replace;
- it may not have been possible to completely stabilise airway, breathing and circulation.

Equipment and staff

Due to the possible dangers associated with patient transfer, potential complications will have to be considered and plans drawn up. All necessary equipment to monitor the patient and effectively manage airway, breathing and circulation must accompany the patient along with appropriately skilled staff. The Intensive Care Society has set national standards for the transfer of the critically ill adult (Intensive Care Society 2002).

Communication and documentation

Communication between the transfer team and the receiving unit/department is paramount. Those receiving the patient need to be informed as to why and when the transfer is happening. The information required prior to transfer should include personal details of the patient, past medical history and reason for transfer. The nature of the patient's clinical condition must also be communicated so that staff at the receiving end can prepare the bed space accordingly.

It is generally good practice to have clear written summaries of events that have taken place but in the case of a patient transfer, it is essential. All relevant notes, scans, results and charts should be made available to the receiving unit along with clear summaries of what has taken place. Cardiac arrest audit forms should be completed after resuscitation events, to allow analysis of where/when arrests are happening, their management and outcome. These are usually returned to the hospital resuscitation officer.

Table 12.5 Levels of classification.

Level 0	Needs met by normal ward care within an acute hospital
Level 1	Needs can be met on acute ward with advice and support from critical care team
Level 2	Requiring detailed observation or intervention due to single failing organ system
Level 3	Requiring advanced ventilatory support together with support of more than one organ system

Definitive placement: where should the patient be managed?

The level of life support required will determine the placement of the patient after a cardiac arrest. A classification of critical care patients has been published by the Department of Health (DoH 2000) as part of a review of critical care services (see Table 12.5).

Rarely will post-arrest patients be anything other than level 2 or 3 unless they either have a 'do not attempt resuscitation' (DNAR) order made or have active treatment withdrawn. Patients who have cardiac disease will usually be cared for in a coronary care unit (CCU) even if they require complex management. As stated in the classification, intensive therapy units (ITU) are for those who need ventilation and/or have multi-system failure.

PREDICTION OF OUTCOME

Return of spontaneous circulation is obviously a favourable outcome from cardiac arrest but significant numbers of these patients do not survive to hospital discharge. It would be advantageous, for both the patient and their relatives, if it were possible to predict in the immediate post-resuscitation phases whether or not long-term survival was likely or even possible.

It would be unethical to deny patients ongoing care if survival was possible so any method that predicts outcome must be entirely reliable. No tests currently exist to determine outcome in the first few hours (Resuscitation Council UK and ERC 2000). Various types of tests and investigations are under review, including blood tests (levels of S-100 protein) and assessment of activity in the brain (electroencephalograph, EEG). Assessment at three days is of far greater reliability than immediately after circulation is restored.

Therapeutic hypothermia

Recently published research has confirmed that mild hypothermia in the 24 hours following an out-of-hospital VF arrest is beneficial to neurological function (Bernard *et al.* 2002). The study subjects who were cooled to 34°C had a significantly better neurological performance than those in the control group who were not cooled. This has led the International Liaison Committee on Resuscitation to issue a statement that unconscious adult survivors of out-of-hospital VF arrest should be cooled to 32–34°C for 12–24 hours (Nolan *et al.* 2003). The statement also suggests that cooling may assist neurological recovery from arrests in hospital or from those with other presenting rhythms.

CARE OF PATIENT'S RELATIVES

Breaking bad news

The issue of breaking bad news to relatives is extremely important and should be undertaken by a senior and experienced member of staff. Conversations of this nature should take place in a quiet room without interruption. Relatives must be allowed time to reflect on the news and to ask any questions they wish. The news may be devastating even if the arrest had occurred after a lengthy and serious period of illness. Several sensitive issues may need to be broached with the relatives, such as whether or not a post mortem is required and the possibility of organ donation (Department for Work and Pensions 2003).

Post mortem

If the cause of death cannot be established or the doctors wish to know more about the cause of death, the coroner may require that funeral arrangements are delayed until a post mortem has been performed. The consent of relatives is not needed but they are entitled to be represented at the examination by a doctor.

Organ donation

If the resuscitation has failed but there is a possibility that the patient's organs or tissue are suitable for donation, the transplant team needs to be involved. Likewise, if the deceased patient had expressed a wish for their organs to be donated, the transplant co-ordinator should be contacted as soon as possible. Should a family member be present, they will be consulted about taking this forward.

The following organs are usually taken from donors who have been certified brain dead but who are ventilated in an ICU.

• Kidneys
• Heart
• Lungs
• Liver
• Pancreas

The following can be removed up to the following times after death.

• Corneas – up to 24 hours
• Skin – up to 24 hours
• Bone – up to 36 hours
• Heart valves – up to 72 hours

Spiritual needs/last offices

Those relatives with specific religious or spiritual beliefs may request contact with a priest or representative of a particular faith. The hospital chaplaincy can help to organise contact. These contacts are not only comforting for relatives but are useful and sometimes necessary as certain faiths have strict requirements as to what happens to the body immediately after death.

CARE OF THE STAFF

Cardiac arrests, particularly on wards where they happen infrequently, can have implications for staff. It is essential that those involved with these extremely stressful situations are given the opportunity for discussion afterwards. They may find it useful to talk through the event and to have questions and concerns addressed. There are often feelings of guilt ('I should have got help sooner') or anger ('Why wasn't the patient allowed to die with dignity?'). These feelings may subside if an honest discussion takes place. For very unexpected and traumatic situations, counselling services or even clinical psychologists may assist staff in coming to terms with these events.

REVIEW OF LEARNING

❏ A structured assessment using the 'A–E' model followed by monitoring supports the recognition of and response to any further cardiac arrests.

❏ Common monitoring includes capnography and arterial pressure monitoring.

❏ Investigations will often include 12-lead ECG, blood tests, arterial blood gases, chest X-ray.

❏ Casualties should be stabilised prior to transfer.

❏ Relatives and staff will require support in the post-resuscitation phase.

Case study

In the week following major surgery, the patient develops signs of dehydration and evidence of worsening infection. The patient subsequently suffers an episode of pulseless electrical activity (PEA) cardiac arrest. The post-arrest team must take into account the management of both potential hypovolaemia and sepsis.

Using the A–E model, discuss what you would monitor in such a patient.

- Airway – look, listen and feel for signs of airway obstruction, ensure airway remains patent potentially using positioning, suction and simple devices.
- Breathing – gauge whether breathing is effective, checking rate and depth, monitor signs of decreased respiratory effort and effects of inadequate oxygenation such as changing heart rate, falling oxygen saturation.

- Circulation – assess signs of adequate circulation by monitoring heart rate, pulse volume, blood pressure, capillary refill, peripheral temperature.
- Disability – monitor level of consciousness using the Glasgow Coma Scale or AVPU scoring system (see pages 262 & 263).
- Exposure – look at the patient, checking urine output, wounds and drainage. Look for signs of bleeding and infection.

As a team member, discuss which aspects you would consider in planning the care and management of the patient.

To conclusively confirm hypovolaemia, a CVP will be placed. Management of hypovolaemia requires fluid replacement (blood, plasma or crystalloids) while avoiding fluid overload. Sepsis may exacerbate hypovolaemia by vasodilation and capillary leakage.

It is important to remember that this patient's history does not exclude the possibility of an arrest secondary to an MI. The patient is likely to require a period of time on a ventilator in the ITU. This will allow assessment and optimisation of heart function, effective management of any infection and support to other systems such as renal function whilst ensuring adequate hydration and nutrition.

CONCLUSION

A significant proportion of cardiac arrest casualties do regain a spontaneous circulation but do not survive to discharge from hospital. This group requires effective continuing care in the post-resuscitation phase to maximise survival chances. Complex management may be necessary alongside careful observation and a series of investigations before the patient is stabilised. If patient transfer is required, only those with experience and expertise must be involved. It is also important to remember that, following a resuscitation event, both the patient's relatives and members of staff may need emotional support.

REFERENCES

Bernard, S., Gray, T., Buist, M. *et al.*, the HACA Study Group (2002) Mild therapeutic hypothermia to improve the neurologic outcome after cardiac arrest. *New England Journal of Medicine* **346**, 549–54.

Department of Health (2000) *Comprehensive Critical Care – A Review of Adult Critical Care Services.* Department of Health, London.

Department for Work and Pensions (2003) *What to Do after a Death in England and Wales – A Guide to What You Must Do and the Help You Can Get.* Department for Work and Pensions, London.

Driscoll, P., Brown, T., Gwinnutt, C. & Wardle, T. (1997) *A Simple Guide to Blood Gas Analysis.* BMJ Books, London.

Gwinnutt, C., Columb, M. & Harris, R. (2000) Outcome after cardiac arrest in hospitals: effect of 1997 guidelines. *Resuscitation* **47**, 125–35.

Howell, M. (2002) The correct use of pulse oximetry in measuring oxygen status. *Professional Nurse* **17** (7), 416–18.

Intensive Care Society (2002) *Guidelines for the Transfer of the Critically Ill Adult*, 2nd edn. Available online at: www.ics.ac.uk/downloads/icstransport2002mem.pdf.

Langhelle, A., Tyvold, S.S., Lexow, K., Hapnes, S.A., Sunde, K. & Steen, P.A. (2003) In-hospital factors associated with improved outcome after out-of-hospital cardiac arrest. A comparison between four regions in Norway. *Resuscitation* **56**, 247–63.

Moore, T. (2004) Pulse oximetry. In: Moore, T. & Woodrow, P. (eds) *High Dependency Nursing Care.* Routledge, London.

Nolan, J.P., Morley, P.T., Vanden Hoek, T.L., Hickey, R.W., the ALS Task Force (2003) Therapeutic hypothermia after cardiac arrest. An advisory statement by the Advanced Life Support Task Force of the International Liaison Committee on Resuscitation. *Resuscitation* **57**, 231–5.

Resuscitation Council UK (2000) *Advanced Life Support Course Provider Manual*, 4th edn. Resuscitation Council UK, London.

Schnell, H. & Puntillo, K. (2001) *Critical Care Nursing Secrets.* Hanley & Belfus Inc, Philadelphia.

Woodrow, P. (2004) Central venous pressure and cardiac output studies. In: Moore, T. & Woodrow, P. (eds) *High Dependency Nursing Care.* Routledge, London.

Special Circumstances   **13**

INTRODUCTION

The universal algorithm provides a sequence of actions for the management of cardiac arrest. There are circumstances, however, in which the team may need to modify its approach to meet the needs of the individual victim. Recognising premonitory signs and responding with prompt treatment may prevent cardiac arrest in these situations. A large proportion of cardiac arrests in younger people who do not have co-existing cardiac disease are due to special circumstances. It is essential to provide early and effective resuscitation to offer the best chance of survival. The circumstances covered in this chapter are:

- anaphylaxis;
- asthma;
- drowning;
- electrocution;
- hypothermia;
- poisoning and drug overdose;
- pregnancy.

AIMS

This chapter discusses how cardiopulmonary resuscitation attempts should be modified in special circumstances.

LEARNING OUTCOMES

At the end of the chapter the reader should be able to:

❏ recognise special circumstances that may require *modification in resuscitation techniques*;

❏ respond to *special emergency situations* appropriately;

❏ discuss *modifications in basic and advanced life support* to meet the needs of the individual casualty and their specific circumstances.

ANAPHYLAXIS

The annual incidence of anaphylaxis is increasing and probably associated with a significant rise in the prevalence of allergic disease over the last two or three decades. Anaphylactic reactions vary in severity and progress may be rapid, slow or (unusually) biphasic. In rare cases, manifestations may be delayed by a few hours (adding to diagnostic difficulty) or persist for more than 24 hours (Resuscitation Council UK 2002). Table 13.1 offers a list of possible causes of anaphylaxis.

Recognising anaphylaxis

Patients with anaphylaxis may present clinically with varying degrees of angio-oedema, urticaria, dyspnoea and hypotension, although death from acute irreversible asthma or laryngeal oedema with few generalised manifestations is possible. Other

Table 13.1 Possible causes of anaphylaxis.

Insect stings, drugs, contrast media, some foods (milk, eggs, fish and shellfish)	Most common causes of anaphylaxis
Peanut and nut allergies	Recognised as particularly dangerous
Aspirin, non-steroidal anti-inflammatory agents, parenteral penicillins and vaccines	Notorious causes of anaphylaxis
Beta-blockers	May increase the incidence and severity of anaphylaxis and antagonise the response to epinephrine

symptoms include rhinitis, conjunctivitis, abdominal pain, vomiting, diarrhoea and a sense of impending doom. The skin colour often changes and the patient may appear either flushed or pale. Cardiovascular collapse is caused by vasodilation and loss of plasma from the blood compartment into the tissues. It is a common clinical manifestation, especially in response to intravenous drugs or stings. Any cardiac dysfunction is due principally to hypotension or, rarely, to an underlying disease or to intravenous administration of epinephrine.

Responding to anaphylaxis

A wide range of possible presentations and clinical signs and symptoms may make it difficult to diagnose anaphylaxis. It is important to undertake a full history and examination as soon as possible. A history of previous allergies as well as the recent incident is vital. Special attention should be given to skin condition (colour, presence of rashes), pulse rate, blood pressure, respiratory rate and auscultation of the chest. A peak flow should also be measured and recorded if possible (Resuscitation Council UK 2002).

Epinephrine (adrenaline) is considered the most important drug for any severe anaphylactic reaction (see Chapter 10). It works by reversing peripheral vasodilation and reducing oedema. It also dilates the airways, increases the force of myocardial contraction and suppresses histamine release. Epinephrine works best when administered early after the onset of the reaction. It is safe when given intramuscularly but does have some risk when given intravenously (Resuscitation Council UK 2002).

Epinephrine injection devices are available for home use. These are currently known as the Epipen (or Anapen) and the Epipen Jr (or Anapen Junior) and can be injected as 300 µg or 150 µg respectively (Resuscitation Council UK 2002). The drug may be given before medical help is available.

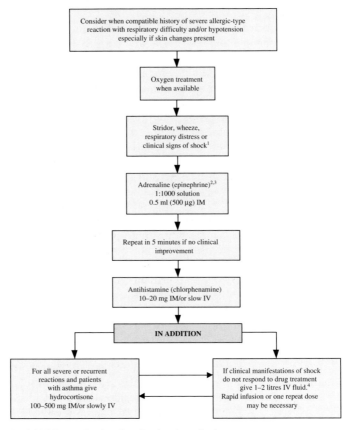

1. An inhaled beta₂-agonist such as salbutamol may be used as an adjunctive measure if bronchospasm is severe and does not respond rapidly to other treatment.

2. If profound shock judged **immediately** life threatening give CPR/ALS if necessary. Consider **slow** IV adrenaline (epinephrine) 1:10 000 solution. This is **hazardous** and is recommended only for an experienced practitioner who can also obtain IV access without delay. Note the different strength of adrenaline (epinephrine) that may be required for IV use.

3. If adults are treated with an Epipen, the 300 μg will usually be sufficient. A second dose may be required. Half doses of adrenaline (epinephrine) may be safer for patients on amitriptyline, imipramine or beta-blocker.

4. A crystalloid may be safer than a colloid.

Fig. 13.1 Anaphylactic reactions. Treatment algorithm for adults by first medical responders (reprinted with permission from the Resuscitation Council UK).

Immediate treatment (see Figure 13.1)

- Position – all casualties should recline in a comfortable position. Lying flat with or without the legs elevated may be helpful if the casualty is hypotensive but unhelpful if there are breathing difficulties.
- The likely allergen should be removed if possible (i.e. stop drug infusion or blood transfusion).
- Oxygen – high-flow oxygen (10–15 l/min) should be administered as soon as possible.
- Airway management – airway obstruction may develop rapidly if there is soft tissue swelling. It is important to consider early tracheal intubation and have the proper equipment readily available.
- Basic and advanced life support – if the casualty is in cardiac arrest, cardiopulmonary resuscitation should be performed according to standard basic and advanced life support guidelines (refer to Chapters 5 and 6).
- Epinephrine (adrenaline) – epinephrine should be administered intramuscularly to all patients with clinical signs of shock, airway swelling or definite breathing difficulty (Resuscitation Council UK 2002). Inspiratory stridor, wheezing, cyanosis, pronounced tachycardia and decreased capillary filling are likely signs of a severe reaction.
- For adults, a dose of 0.5 ml epinephrine 1:1000 solution (500 µg) should be administered intramuscularly. This should be repeated after about five minutes if there is no clinical improvement or if the patient deteriorates after the initial treatment, especially if hypotension causes the level of consciousness to become or remain impaired. In some cases several doses may be needed, particularly if improvement is transient.
- Intravenous administration of epinephrine should only be given in a dilution of at least 1:10000 (**never** 1:1000). It must be reserved for patients with profound shock that is immediately life threatening and for special indications, for example during anaesthesia. Heart rate and ECG monitoring are essential when giving an epinephrine infusion.
- Antihistamines – an antihistamine (chlorphenamine) should be administered to block the effects of histamine release

(American Heart Association (AHA) and International Liaison Committee on Resuscitation (ILCOR) 2000). The drug may cause hypotension. It must be given by either slow intravenous injection or intramuscular injection. The adult dose is 10–20 mg intramuscularly.

- Corticosteroids – hydrocortisone (as sodium succinate) should be administered after severe attacks to help avert late sequelae. The dose of hydrocortisone for adults is 100–500 mg and must be given by slow intravenous or intramuscular injection (AHA & ILCOR 2000).
- Fluid administration – a rapid infusion of 1–2 litres of fluid (such as normal saline) may be needed if severe hypotension persists after drug treatment.

Further management
- Patients with even moderately severe attacks of anaphylaxis should be warned of the possibility of an early recurrence of symptoms and in some circumstances should be kept under observation for up to 24 hours.
- If possible, the allergen should be identified and the patient should be advised to avoid future exposure.
- Patients at high risk of anaphylaxis may wish to carry their own epinephrine syringe and wear a 'Medic-alert' type bracelet.
- All patients who have suffered a severe reaction should be referred to a specialist allergy clinic for further investigation and assessment.

ACUTE SEVERE ASTHMA
It is important to differentiate routine asthma care from that in acute severe asthma. This section will focus on acute or near-fatal asthma, a condition that is largely reversible so related deaths should be considered avoidable. Interventions are aimed at preventing respiratory and secondary cardiac arrest (AHA & ILCOR 2000, Scottish Intercollegiate Guidelines Network (SIGN) & British Thoracic Society (BTS) 2003).

Most deaths related to acute severe asthma occur outside hospital. Contributing factors include:

- patients and their relatives seek medical care late because they do not understand or recognise the severity of the attack;
- emergency services or medical professionals may be slow to respond;
- patients with less severe asthma attacks may seek emergency care but after treatment are discharged home and deteriorate further.

Cardiac arrest may occur in patients with severe asthma as a result of any of the following:

- hypoxia from mucus plugging or severe bronchospasm;
- cardiac arrhythmias from hypoxia or as a side-effect of beta agonists and aminophylline;
- tension pneumothorax.

Recognising acute severe asthma
- Silent chest
- Cyanosis
- Weak or ineffective respiratory effort
- Fatigue, exhaustion, confusion or even coma
- Associated bradycardia and hypotension
- Arterial blood gases will indicate hypoxia, acidaemia, normal or high carbon dioxide tension

Responding to acute severe asthma
- All exacerbations of asthma must be treated aggressively to prevent near-fatal asthma and cardiac arrest. Patients should be cared for in a critical care environment with full monitoring and observation.
- Oxygen – high-flow oxygen (10–15 l/min) should be administered as soon as possible.
- First-line therapy – inhaled beta agonists are recommended. Nebulised salbutamol, 5 mg in 5 ml of normal saline, should be administered with oxygen or alternatively 4–6 puffs through a metered dose inhaler with a holding chamber (SIGN & BTS 2003).
- Corticosteroid therapy – either oral or intravenous corticosteroids should be given in the first 30 minutes (SIGN & BTS 2003).

- Other therapies – inhaled anticholinergics, intravenous aminophylline, intravenous magnesium sulphate or Heliox may be used if patients fail to respond to other treatments (SIGN & BTS 2003).
- Fluid replacement – patients with severe acute asthma will often be dehydrated and benefit from intravenous fluid replacement.
- Basic and advanced life support – standard guidelines for basic and advanced life support should be followed.
- It may be difficult to ventilate the patient's lungs because of high airway resistance. Ventilation with a bag-valve-face-mask may predispose the patient to gastric inflation. Tracheal intubation should be performed as early as possible.
- The patient may have a hyperinflated chest, making chest compressions difficult or impossible. To overcome this, allow a prolonged expiratory time between breaths (AHA & ILCOR 2000).
- Any arrhythmias should be treated according to the current advanced life support (ALS) guidelines.

DROWNING

Drowning is defined as a process resulting in primary respiratory impairment from submersion or immersion in a liquid medium, usually water. This prevents the casualty from breathing air. The casualty may live or die after this process but whatever the outcome, the individual has been involved in a drowning incident (Idris *et al.* 2003).

Recognising drowning

- Hypoxia and hypercarbia are important consequences of drowning. The outcome will largely depend on how long the patient was hypoxic. Therefore oxygenation, ventilation and perfusion should be restored as rapidly as possible.
- Hypothermia may occur in water 25°C or less and may be another factor to consider.
- Drowning is sometimes precipitated by an injury or medical condition. It is important to recognise and report this if known. Examples may include (Idris *et al.* 2003):

—seizure;

—level of consciousness and/or motor function impaired by drugs, alcohol or hypothermia;

—circulatory arrest (e.g. ventricular fibrillation or pulseless electrical activity);

—trauma;

—unconsciousness from any other cause.

Responding to drowning

- Resuscitation efforts should start at the scene if the casualty is to have the best chance of survival and full neurological recovery (AHA & ILCOR 2000). Basic life support should be commenced (refer to Chapter 5). It makes no difference if the accident occurred in fresh or salt water.

- It is important to be aware of personal safety and minimise danger when reaching and recovering the casualty. Attempt to keep the casualty horizontal. Vertical removal from water may cause circulatory collapse (AHA & ILCOR 2000).

- Resuscitation should start unless there are obvious lethal injuries, putrefaction or rigor mortis.

- If there is a possibility of spinal cord injury, such as after diving into shallow water, the spine should be immobilised during recovery. The jaw thrust should be used to open the airway, rather than head tilt, chin lift.

- Rescue breathing should begin as quickly as possible. It can be attempted once the rescuer can stand in the water or the casualty is on land. If it is difficult to perform mouth-to-mouth ventilation while supporting the casualty's head in the water, mouth-to-nose ventilation is an acceptable alternative.

- The airway should be inspected and any debris removed. It is **not** necessary to remove water from the airway before starting BLS. Attempting to tip the casualty head down will not help remove water and may cause vomiting and aspiration.

- Vomiting is a common occurrence in submersion events. The person's head should be turned to the side. Suction should be used to remove vomitus. Early tracheal intubation will help prevent aspiration of vomit.

- It may be difficult to palpate a pulse if the casualty is cold. If no signs of circulation are present, chest compressions should be started as soon as possible. Do not attempt chest compressions while the casualty is still in water.

- Successful resuscitation with full neurological recovery has been reported in casualties with prolonged submersion in cold water therefore life support should continue for a longer period than usual (AHA & ILCOR 2000).

Advanced life support

- Advanced life support should be initiated without delay as necessary.
- Every drowning casualty should be transferred to a medical facility, even if only minimal resuscitation was necessary and the casualty regained consciousness. These patients are at high risk for developing other problems such as adult respiratory distress syndrome (ARDS), circulatory collapse or pulmonary oedema (Resuscitation Council UK 2000).
- The guidelines for hypothermia should be followed if the patient is hypothermic (<35°C).
- The insertion of a nasogastric tube will aid in decompressing and emptying the stomach.

ELECTROCUTION

Electrocution may occur as a result of domestic or industrial electricity or lightning strike. Adults are mostly likely to experience electrical injury in the workplace, while children are more at risk at home. There are approximately 1000 deaths worldwide every year from lightning strike (Auerbach 1995). Injuries may range from a transient, unpleasant sensation from contact with a low current to cardiac arrest from exposure to high voltage or current. The severity of electrical injury is also dependent on whether the current is alternating (a.c.) or direct (d.c.), magnitude of the energy delivered, resistance to current flow, pathway of current through the casualty and the area and duration of electrical contact (Lederer *et al*. 1999).

Recognising electrocution

- Contact with alternating current (a.c.) often causes tetanic contraction of skeletal muscle. Furthermore, casualties may not be able to release themselves from the source of electricity and respiratory arrest may also occur. The alternating current may also cause ventricular fibrillation.

- Extensive tissue damage may occur along the electrical current pathway. A transthoracic (hand-to-hand) pathway is more likely to be fatal than a vertical (hand-to-foot) or straddle (foot-to-foot) pathway.

- Asystole or ventricular fibrillation will most likely be present after a lightning strike as a result of a massive, direct shock that depolarises the entire myocardium. Respiratory muscle paralysis may also occur, leading to respiratory arrest. Secondary cardiac arrest may happen if respiratory arrest is not treated promptly and effectively.

- Immediately after any type of electrocution, the casualty may have respiratory or cardiac failure or both. The casualty may appear apnoeic or mottled or become unconscious. The casualty may also have contact burns at the point of entry and exit. It is essential to use the ABC approach in the initial assessment (refer to Chapter 2).

Responding to electrocution

- Safety – the rescuer must be certain that he or she will not be in danger while attempting to rescue the casualty. Any power source should be turned off. Rescuers should also be aware that high-voltage electricity can 'arc' and conduct through the ground for up to a few metres around the casualty.

- Standard basic and advanced life support should be started as soon as possible.

- Airway – electrical burns around the face and neck may cause extensive soft tissue oedema that can lead to airway obstruction. Early intubation may be necessary. Head and spine trauma may also occur with electrocution. Spine immobilisation should be carried out until a thorough evaluation is made.

- Circulation – the commonest initial arrhythmia after high voltage a.c. shock is ventricular fibrillation. This may be due to the alternating current acting on the myocardium during the vulnerable repolarisation phase, also known as R-on-T phenomenon (Lederer *et al*. 1999). This should be treated promptly with attempted defibrillation following standard protocols. Asystole is the commonest arrhythmia following high-voltage d.c. shock due to the massive, direct current that can depolarise the entire myocardium (Lederer *et al.* 1999). Treatment of asystole and any other arrhythmias should follow standard protocols.

- Other considerations – burns may occur from shoes or smouldering clothing. These items should be removed as soon as possible. Aggressive fluid therapy may also be required if there is serious tissue damage.

- Survivors of electrical injury should be monitored in hospital if they have a history of cardiorespiratory problems or have suffered loss of consciousness, cardiac arrest, ECG abnormalities or soft tissue damage and burns (AHA & ILCOR 2000).

HYPOTHERMIA

Hypothermia occurs when the body core temperature falls below 35°C. It can happen when people with normal thermoregulation are exposed to cold environments or after immersion in cold water. In someone with impaired thermoregulation, hypothermia may occur from a mild cold insult. Hypothermia occurs in all four seasons and casualty presentation does not seem to depend only on ambient temperature (AHA & ILCOR 2000).

Recognising hypothermia

- Clinical history and examination of the casualty may indicate hypothermia but it is confirmed using a low-reading thermometer to measure core temperature (see Table 13.2). An oesophageal, rectal or tympanic thermometer should be used.

- Casualties may appear to be clinically dead because the brain and heart function have slowed significantly and signs of life are very difficult to detect.

- Hypothermia can actually have a protective effect on the brain. Mild hypothermia may improve neurological function after a VF arrest (Nolan *et al.* 2003).

- Resuscitation should not be withheld based on clinical presentation. Also, once resuscitation attempts have started, the team should continue until the casualty has been rewarmed. This may mean a prolonged resuscitation.

Table 13.2 Classification of hypothermia.

Classification of hypothermia	Temperature (°C)
Mild	35–32°
Moderate	32–30°
Severe	Below 30°

Responding to hypothermia

- Preventing cardiac arrest – if the casualty is extremely cold but still has a perfusing rhythm, interventions should focus on assessment and support of airway, breathing and circulation, preventing further heat loss, rewarming and careful transport to a hospital.
- The casualty should be removed from the cold environment.
- Cold, wet clothing should be removed when it is practical. If the temperature is less than 25°C or there is wind, it may be better to leave wet garments on and wrap the casualty in blankets to avoid increased exposure (Auerbach 1995).
- Blankets and insulating equipment may be used to protect against further heat loss.
- Rough movement and activity can precipitate VF and should be avoided.
- Urgent procedures such as tracheal intubation or insertion of central venous catheters should be done gently and carefully while monitoring the heart rhythm closely.
- Core temperature and cardiac rhythm must be monitored.

Rewarming

- Casualties with a core temperature of less than 34°C should be rewarmed (AHA & ILCOR 2000).
- Rewarming should occur at a rate that correlates with the rate of onset of hypothermia, although this may be difficult to determine (see Table 13.3).

Basic life support modifications
- Basic life support (BLS) should be initiated according to the guidelines (described in Chapter 5).
- Hypothermia slows breathing and causes peripheral vasoconstriction. For this reason breathing may be shallow and the pulse difficult to feel. It may be necessary to assess breathing and pulse for a period of 30–45 seconds to confirm arrest (AHA & ILCOR 2000).
- The ventilation:compression ratio (15:2) should be the same as for casualties with a normal temperature. Hypothermia can make the chest wall feel stiff and ventilation and compressions more difficult. The lungs should be ventilated with enough volume to cause the chest to rise visibly. The rescuer should aim to achieve a compression depth of 4–5 cm.
- BLS should continue until the casualty has been rewarmed.

Advanced life support modifications
- Advanced life support should be initiated according to the universal algorithm (see Chapter 6).

Table 13.3 Definitions of rewarming.

Passive rewarming	Achieved with blankets and a warm room. This method alone will not be effective for patients in cardiac arrest or severely hypothermic	All hypothermic patients
Active external warming	Heating devices (e.g. bair huggar), warm bath water or radiant heat. Use caution since some heating devices can cause tissue injury	Mild and moderate hypothermia
Active internal warming	Warmed, humidified oxygen, peritoneal, gastric, pleural or bladder lavage with warm fluid (40°C), intravenous administration of warmed fluids (e.g. normal saline). Follow local hospital policy	Severe hypothermia

- Arrhythmias – procedures such as endotracheal intubation can cause VF. However, this should not be withheld when urgently indicated.
- Defibrillation – if the core temperature is <30°C, VF may not respond to the first three shocks. Further shocks should be delayed until the patient's body core temperature is >30°C. Continue CPR during this time (AHA & ILCOR 2000).
- Drugs and drug administration – where possible, a central or large proximal vein should be cannulated. The casualty with hypothermia may not respond to cardioactive drugs. Drug metabolism is reduced and this may lead to a build-up of drugs in the system. Epinephrine (adrenaline) and other drugs are generally withheld until the temperature is >30°C. Once this target is reached, the intervals between doses should be doubled and the lowest recommended dose given. Once the temperature is near normal, standard drug protocols can be used (AHA & ILCOR 2000).

Death is not confirmed until the casualty is warm or attempts to raise core temperature have failed. A full recovery without neurological deficit may be possible even after prolonged hypothermic cardiac arrest (Resuscitation Council UK 2000).

POISONING AND DRUG INTOXICATION

Poisoning is a leading cause of death in people less than 40 years old and is also the commonest cause of non-traumatic coma in this age group. Hospital admission is usually the result of self-poisoning with therapeutic or recreational drugs. Accidental poisoning is more common in children (AHA & ILCOR 2000).

Recognising poisoning and drug intoxication

- Death is commonly caused by airway obstruction and respiratory arrest secondary to a decreased level of consciousness. Recognising airway and breathing problems should be a high priority.

- In an unconscious or arrested casualty, it may be difficult to determine whether the cause was poisoning. This must be excluded as a possible reason for the coma.

Responding to poisoning and drug intoxication

- Management of the casualty with self-poisoning (overdose) should focus on airway, breathing and circulation support to prevent cardiorespiratory arrest while waiting for drug elimination from the body. Basic and advanced life support should proceed according to the standard guidelines when there is cardiac arrest (Chapters 5 and 6).
- Airway and breathing – basic airway opening manoeuvres should be used. If the patient is not breathing, the lungs should be ventilated using a pocket mask or bag-valve-facemask and the highest possible concentration of oxygen. It is especially important to avoid any mouth-to-mouth contact in the presence of toxins such as cyanide, hydrogen sulphide, corrosives and organophosphates (Resuscitation Council UK 2000).
- Early intubation – pulmonary aspiration of gastric contents is highly likely after poisoning. Early intubation is recommended in unconscious casualties who are unable to protect their own airway (AHA & ILCOR 2000).
- It is important to identify the poison as soon as possible after resuscitation has started. Relatives, friends and emergency medical system crews may be able to provide information. The casualty should also be examined for needle puncture marks, tablet residues, signs of corrosion in the mouth or skin breakdown from lying in one position during prolonged coma.
- The TOXBASE (www.spib.axl.co.uk), co-ordinated by the Edinburgh Centre of the National Poisons Information Service (NPIS), can be accessed for specialist help on specific therapeutic measures.
- The emphasis with any poisoning should be on intensive supportive therapy, correction of hypoxia, acid–base and electrolyte disorders. The following specific therapeutic measures may be useful (AHA & ILCOR 2000).

—Gastric lavage followed by activated charcoal – only recommended within one hour of ingesting the poison. Tracheal intubation should precede this intervention.

—Haemodialysis or haemoperfusion may increase drug elimination.

—Specific antidotes may be effective in certain situations, as shown in Table 13.4.

Table 13.4 A guide to poisons and possible antidotes or therapeutic measures.

Poison	Specific antidote or possible therapeutic measure
Paracetamol	N-acetylcysteine
Benzodiazapines (midazolam, diazepam, lorazepam)	Flumazenil
Tricyclic antidepressants	No specific antidote but administration of sodium bicarbonate may provide some myocardial protection and prevent arrhythmias
Opioids	Naloxone – the duration of action is shorter than the duration of most opioids and repeated doses may be needed
Cocaine toxicity	No specific antidote but small doses of intravenous benzodiazepines are effective first-line agents. Nitrates may be used as second-line therapy for myocardial ischaemia. Labetalol (alpha- and beta-blocker) is helpful for tachycardia and hypertensive emergencies
Digoxin	Digoxin-specific Fab antibodies (Digi-bind)
Organophosphate insecticides	High-dose atropine
Cyanide	Sodium nitrite, sodium thiosulphate or dicobalt edetate

PREGNANCY

Pregnancy creates a unique situation because there are two people to resuscitate. The emphasis must be on effective life support for the mother and this will in turn optimise fetal outcome. There may be many different reasons for cardiac arrest in pregnant women and it is most commonly related to changes and events that occur around the time of delivery (AHA & ILCOR 2000).

Recognising an emergency in pregnancy

Causes of maternal cardiac arrest may include haemorrhage, pulmonary embolism, amniotic fluid embolism, placental abruption, eclampsia and drug toxicity. Physiological changes occur during pregnancy and these must be considered during an emergency.

- Gastric emptying is delayed after the first trimester of pregnancy and there may be an increased risk of pulmonary aspiration of gastric contents.
- Anatomical changes such as breast enlargement, obesity of the neck and glottic oedema may make airway management difficult. Also, in later stages of pregnancy, the diaphragm is splinted by a large uterus and higher than normal inflation pressures may be needed to achieve effective ventilation.
- Cardiovascular problems may occur because the uterus presses down against the inferior vena cava and reduces or blocks blood flow to the heart.

Responding

- An obstetrician and neonatologist should be involved as early as possible (Resuscitation Council UK 2000).
- All principles of basic and advanced life support apply to the pregnant woman.
- Cardiac arrest may be prevented with early intervention. Cardiac output and venous return may be improved by relieving pressure on the inferior vena cava and aorta (AHA & ILCOR 2000). This can be achieved by:

—placing sandbags, pillows or a purpose-made (Cardiff) wedge under the patient's right buttock and lower back;

—placing the patient in the left lateral position;

—manually moving the uterus to the left.

- Chest compression is performed in the standard way. The rescuer should be aware that it may be more difficult because of breast hypertrophy and splinting of the diaphragm.
- Arrhythmias should be treated according to standard protocols.

Emergency caesarean section is recommended after five minutes of unsuccessful resuscitation to improve the chances of both fetal and maternal survival (Resuscitation Council UK 2000).

REVIEW OF LEARNING

❏ Special circumstances may occur that require the team to modify its approach to resuscitation.

❏ Recognising and responding early may prevent cardiac arrest in special circumstances.

❏ Anaphylaxis is increasingly common. Epinephrine (adrenaline) given intramuscularly is considered the most important drug for any severe anaphylactic reaction.

❏ Acute severe asthma is largely reversible and related deaths should be considered avoidable.

❏ Asthma exacerbations must be treated aggressively with oxygen, inhaled beta agonists and corticosteroid therapy.

❏ Hypoxia and hypercarbia are consequences of drowning. Oxygenation, ventilation and perfusion should be restored as rapidly as possible.

❏ Successful resuscitation with full neurological recovery has been reported in casualties with prolonged submersion in cold water therefore life support should continue for a longer period than usual.

❏ Electrocution may occur from an alternating current (a.c.) or direct current (d.c.). Asystole and VF are common arrhythmias that should be treated according to the universal algorithm.

❏ Mild hypothermia may improve neurological function after a VF arrest.

❏ Rewarming the hypothermic casualty should occur at a rate that correlates with the rate of onset of hypothermia.

❏ Death in poisoning is commonly caused by airway obstruction and respiratory arrest secondary to a decreased level of consciousness. Recognising airway and breathing problems should be a high priority.

❏ Pregnancy creates a unique situation because there are two people to resuscitate. The emphasis must be on effective life support for the mother and this will in turn optimise fetal outcome.

❏ Cardiac output and venous return may be improved by relieving pressure on the inferior vena cava and aorta in the pregnant casualty.

Case study

Fred Hughes is a 70-year-old man admitted to the hospital for treatment of community-acquired pneumonia. A few minutes after the first dose of intravenous benzylpenicillin, Fred complains of feeling sick, vomits and becomes unresponsive.

What do you suspect is happening? What other signs and symptoms might be present?

It is likely that Mr Hughes is having an anaphylactic reaction due to administration of intravenous antibiotic. Specific signs and symptoms to watch out for include varying degrees of angio-oedema, urticaria, dyspnoea and hypotension. The patient may also have rhinitis, conjunctivitis, diarrhoea and a sense of impending doom. The skin colour often changes and the patient may appear either flushed or pale. Cardiovascular collapse is caused by vasodilation and loss of plasma from the blood compartment into the tissues. It is a common clinical manifestation, especially in response to intravenous drugs or stings.

During your physical examination you note that Fred's skin is red and flushed and there is generalised urticaria. His tongue is swollen and he is having difficulty breathing. His heart rate is 120 bpm and his blood pressure is 65/40. **How would you respond to this situation?**

- Call for help.
- Stop the infusion of benzylpenicillin.
- Administer high-flow oxygen (10–15 l/min). Assess the patient for airway obstruction and be prepared with airway adjuncts discussed in Chapter 7.
- Give epinephrine (adrenaline) 1 : 1000 solution 0.5 ml intramuscularly. Alternatively use an Epipen.
- Epinephrine IM may be repeated after about five minutes if there is no clinical improvement or if the patient deteriorates after the initial treatment, especially if hypotension causes the level of consciousness to become or remain impaired.
- Administer an antihistamine (chlorphenamine). It must be given either by slow intravenous injection or by intramuscular injection. The adult dose is 10–20 mg IM.
- Consider administration of hydrocortisone 100–500 mg IM.
- If there are still clinical signs of shock after drug treatment, give 1–2 litres intravenous fluid.

REFERENCES

American Heart Association and International Liaison Committee on Resuscitation (2000) Part 8. Advanced challenges in resuscitation. *Circulation* 102 (suppl I), I217–I252.

Auerbach, P.S. (ed.) (1995) *Wilderness Medicine: Management of Wilderness and Environmental Emergencies*, 3rd edn. Mosby, Philadelphia.

Idris, A.H., Berg, R.A., Bierens, J. *et al.* (2003) Recommended guidelines for uniform reporting of data from drowning: the "Utstein Style". *Resuscitation* **59**, 45–57.

Lederer, W., Wiedermann, F.J., Cerchiari, E. & Baubin, M.A. (1999) Electricity-associated injuries I: outdoor management of current-induced casualties. *Resuscitation* **43**, 69–77.

Nolan, J.P., Morley, P.T., Vanden Hoek, T.L., Hickey, R.W., the ALS Task Force (2003) Therapeutic hypothermia after cardiac arrest. An advisory statement by the Advanced Life Support Task Force of the International Liaison Committee on Resuscitation. *Resuscitation* **57**, 231–5.

Resuscitation Council UK (2000) *Advanced Life Support Course Provider Manual*, 4th edn. Resuscitation Council UK, London.

Resuscitation Council UK (2002) *The Emergency Medical Treatment of Anaphylactic Reactions for First Medical Responders and for Community Nurses*. Available online at: www.resus.org.uk/pages/reaction.htm.

Scottish Intercollegiate Guidelines Network and British Thoracic Society (2003) *British Guideline on the Management of Asthma*. Available online at: www.brit-thoracic.org.uk/sign.

Resuscitation of the Seriously Injured Casualty

14

INTRODUCTION

Trauma is the major cause of morbidity and mortality in otherwise healthy adults, with 3000 people dying and 30000 being injured every day on the world's roads. Trauma is the leading cause of death in the first three decades of life and millions are injured each year and survive. For many, the injury causes temporary pain and inconvenience but for some it leads to disability, chronic pain and a profound change in lifestyle. Preventive public health measures such as safety belts and health and safety laws are the key to decreasing these numbers.

Trauma deaths occur in three peaks.

- Peak 1 refers to 'immediate' deaths at the scene of an accident due to lethal and usually untreatable injuries.
- Peak 2 describes deaths occurring in the first few hours after injury. These early deaths are usually due to airway, breathing and circulation failure or head injury. They may be prevented by early treatment during what is called the *golden hour* of trauma resuscitation.
- Peak 3 deaths occur weeks or months after the injury. These late deaths usually occur in the critical care unit and are due to sepsis and multiple organ failure.

AIMS

This chapter provides a structured approach to the initial resuscitation of the seriously injured casualty.

LEARNING OUTCOMES

At the end of the chapter the reader should be able to:

❏ prepare for *reception* of the seriously injured casualty;
❏ understand the *role of the trauma team*;

❏ understand the *key steps in the initial management* of the seriously injured casualty;
❏ safely *transfer the casualty* for definitive care.

RECEPTION OF THE SERIOUSLY INJURED CASUALTY

The ambulance service will often warn the emergency department of the arrival of a seriously injured casualty. This allows preparation of the resuscitation room and alerting of the trauma team. However, there will always be casualties who arrive unexpectedly with serious injury and therefore the emergency department should be prepared to receive casualties at short notice.

The resuscitation room

The resuscitation room needs to be ready to accept casualties. Drugs and equipment stocks should be checked at the beginning of every shift, using a checklist to ensure items are not missed. Equipment such as defibrillators, oxygen cylinders and suction should be in working order.

THE TRAUMA TEAM

Trauma team members should be ready in the resuscitation room to receive the seriously injured casualty (Gwinnutt & Driscoll 2003). Information received from ambulance control will usually indicate whether the trauma team is required and Table 14.1 lists factors associated with serious injuries. There should be a medical and nursing team leader and the team should include members with the following skills.

Table 14.1 Factors associated with serious injury.

Fall from a height of 4 or more metres
High-speed impact in road traffic accident
Death of other passengers at scene of road accident
Ejection from vehicle
Motorcyclist with no helmet involved in accident
Significant damage to the passenger compartment of vehicle

- Assessment and treatment of the seriously injured.
- Advanced airway skills – this includes the ability to perform a rapid-sequence induction and tracheal intubation.
- Advanced cannulation skills.
- Radiographer for X-ray images.
- Portering.
- Record and timekeeping.
- Team member for liaising with relatives or to accompany relatives if they wish to be present during the resuscitation.

Personal protective equipment (PPE)

Trauma team members need to ensure their personal safety by taking universal precautions. Minimum precautions when dealing with a seriously injured casualty include:

- eye protection
- gloves
- waterproof aprons
- X-ray gowns

All body fluids should be treated as potentially infected. When casualties arrive in the emergency department they will often be dressed and covered in debris that can include glass fragments and other sharp objects and extra precautions are needed for casualties of biological or chemical attack. These casualties require decontamination at the scene of the incident or immediately on arrival to hospital prior to entering the emergency department.

IN-HOSPITAL RESUSCITATION

Successful resuscitation of the seriously injured casualty requires a systematic approach to patient management. The most commonly used system is based on advanced trauma life support (ATLS) course principles developed by the American College of Surgeons in the 1970s (American College of Surgeons 1997). Team members perform a number of tasks simultaneously, with the initial management consisting of three phases:

- primary survey and resuscitation
- secondary survey
- definitive care.

Primary survey and resuscitation

The primary survey identifies and treats life-threatening injuries in the order in which they are most likely to kill the patient. The priorities for recognising and responding are:

- *A*: Airway with cervical spine control
- *B*: Breathing
- *C*: Circulation and haemorrhage control
- *D*: Dysfunction, refers to neurological status
- *E*: Exposure and environment.

A: Airway and cervical spine

It is important that the casualty has a clear airway and adequate oxygenation. The airway is assessed and managed as described in Chapter 7, with the proviso that the cervical spine is protected. A patient who can speak clearly has a clear airway, whereas the unconscious patient may require help with maintaining an open airway and breathing. Snoring, gurgling and stridor can indicate an upper airway obstruction.

A cervical spine injury should be assumed in all patients with severe trauma until it has been excluded. Jaw thrust and airway adjuncts are the preferred methods to open the airway of the unconscious trauma patient.

The cervical spine is immobilised with one of two methods:

- manual in-line stabilisation. A team member holds the casualty's head and neck in the neutral position;
- semi-rigid cervical collar blocks and tape (see Figure 14.1).

Seriously injured patients are at high risk of vomiting and aspiration of gastric contents. Patients with a decreased conscious level and inability to protect their airway require early tracheal intubation which is ideally performed using a rapid-sequence induction (RSI) technique. This requires administration of an intravenous sedative, a fast-onset, short-acting muscle relaxant (suxamethonium) and the application of cricoid pressure. Once the patient is fully sedated and relaxed the trachea is intubated. This requires specialist training (Clancy & Nolan 2002). The head is held using manual in-line stabilisation during tracheal intubation to ensure the cervical spine is not moved. This is preferable to using head blocks and a cervical collar, which can make access and mouth opening difficult.

B: Breathing

All patients must initially be given oxygen at the highest concentration possible. A fully conscious patient who is breathing normally requires a facemask with reservoir and high-flow oxygen (10–15 l/min). A patient who is not breathing will require assistance with breathing using a bag-valve-mask device.

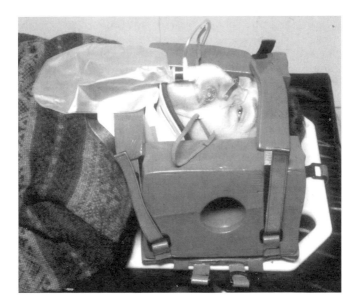

Fig. 14.1 Immobilisation of the cervical spine using collar blocks and straps.

Chest injuries will cause difficulty in breathing and the patient may have a fast or slow respiratory rate and also be hypoxic. The need for oxygen to maintain a normal oxygen saturation also indicates there is a problem. The team leader should look for and treat life-threatening chest injuries in the primary survey. These can be diagnosed clinically and excluded in the primary survey (see Table 14.2). The recognition of and response to these injuries require specialist training.

C: Circulation

'Shock' is defined as inadequate organ perfusion and tissue oxygenation. The recognition of hypovolaemic shock is based on clinical findings: hypotension, tachycardia, tachypnoea, altered conscious level as well as hypothermia, pallor, cool extremities, decreased capillary refill and decreased urine production.

A low blood pressure (hypotension) is assumed to be due to bleeding (haemorrhage) in the injured patient unless proven otherwise. The amount of blood loss after trauma is often poorly assessed and in blunt trauma is usually underestimated. Often large volumes of blood may be hidden in the abdominal and chest cavity. A femoral fracture can be associated with a 2 litre blood loss. This is a large proportion of the blood volume if one considers that the total blood volume of a 70 kg male is 5 litres. Bleeding must therefore be identified and stopped to prevent hypovolaemic shock. Hypovolaemic shock in the adult can be categorised into four stages (I, II, III, IV) based on the amount of blood loss (see Table 14.3).

Capillary refill is measured by pressing a distal digit at heart level for five seconds. A normal capillary return time is less than two seconds. This can be affected by cold weather so it must be interpreted with other signs and symptoms.

The response to hypovolaemic shock is to stop the bleeding and correct the blood volume. Wound bleeding can be stopped by applying direct pressure. Internal blood loss may require rapid transfer to an operating theatre for surgical control of blood loss. Blood volume is restored using intravenous fluids and blood.

Table 14.2 Chest injuries identified and treated in the primary survey.

Injury	Recognition	Response
Tension pneumothorax	Decreased air entry, decreased expansion and hyperresonance to percussion on the side of injury. Trachea deviated away from injured side	Needle thoracocentesis. A large-bore needle is placed in the second intercostal space, midclavicular line to relieve the tension. A chest drain is then inserted
Open pneumothorax	There is a hole in the casualty's chest wall, which sucks on inspiration: 'sucking chest wound'	The hole should be covered with a square waterproof dressing that is taped down on three sides. This stops air being sucked in but allows air to escape through the hole. A chest drain is then inserted
Massive haemothorax	There is bleeding in the chest. The affected side will have decreased expansion and air entry and will be dull to percussion. A large volume of blood can be lost in the chest so the patient may be shocked	Chest drain inserted on injured side. If there is a large amount of blood loss the patient requires immediate surgery to stop the bleeding
Flail chest	This occurs when there are a large number of rib fractures. A portion of the chest wall (flail segment) moves freely. This limits expansion of the lungs on inspiration. The flail segment will not move on chest expansion. The extent of the rib fractures also indicates that the chest has been struck with a large force so there is usually an underlying lung injury (lung contusion)	Oxygen, analgesia to make breathing less painful. Tracheal intubation and controlled ventilation if there is severe lung contusion
Cardiac tamponade	Bleeding around the heart may prevent it pumping effectively. It can occur after blunt or penetrating trauma. The patient will be shocked (low blood pressure) and there may be a wound (between the nipples or shoulder blades). There may be muffled heart sounds and distended neck veins	Pericardiocentesis. A drain is inserted into the pericardial space and any blood around the heart removed. Effective treatment may require an urgent thoracotomy in the emergency room (Rhee *et al.* 2000)

Table 14.3 Categories of hypovolaemic shock.

	I	II	III	IV
Blood loss (litres)	<0.75	0.75–1.5	1.5–2.0	>2.0
Percentage blood loss (%)	<15	15–30	30–40	>40
Heart rate	<100	>100	>120	>140 or low
Systolic BP	Normal	Normal	Decreased	Decreased ++
Diastolic BP	Normal	Raised	Decreased	Decreased ++
Pulse pressure	Normal	Decreased	Decreased	Decreased
Capillary refill	Normal	Delayed	Delayed	Delayed
Skin colour	Normal	Pale	Very pale	Very pale/ cold
Respiratory rate	14–20	20–30	30–40	>35 or low
Mental state	Normal/ anxious	Anxious	Anxious/ confused	Confused/ drowsy
Fluid choice	None/ crystalloid	Crystalloid/ colloid	Blood	Blood

Pulse pressure = systolic BP – diastolic BP

Intravenous access must be established early during the resuscitation. Two large-bore cannulae (14 gauge) should be inserted. At this time blood should be taken for the following investigations:

- full blood count
- urea and electrolytes
- coagulation study
- glucose
- cross-matching
- consider a pregnancy test in females of child-bearing age
- arterial blood gases.

It is pointless giving large amounts of intravenous fluids to a patient who is actively bleeding if no effort is made to stop the blood loss. The role of fluid resuscitation at this stage is to keep the patient alive until there is definitive control of bleeding. As mentioned previously, this requires direct pressure, splinting of fractures or immediate surgery. Failure to stop bleeding results in excessive fluid administration. This can cause increased blood loss as clots may be disrupted at the injury site due to increased blood pressure and dilution of clotting factors and platelets (Revell *et al*. 2003).

The choice of resuscitation fluids is controversial (Nolan 2001). Fluids that could be used include crystalloids (Hartmann's or 0.9% normal saline) and colloids such as gelatins (Gelofusin, Haemaccel), dextrans or starches. Current evidence indicates that there is no real advantage in using the more expensive colloids over cheaper crystalloids for initial fluid management in trauma patients. The volume given should be based on the response in terms of improvements in blood pressure, pulse and conscious level.

The amount and urgency of blood transfusion will depend on the degree of hypovolaemia. In multiple injuries it may be necessary to order 6–10 units of blood. If blood is required immediately, the blood bank will supply group O blood, which has not been grouped or cross-matched to the patient. If it is possible to wait 10–15 minutes, the blood bank can supply group-confirmed blood. This is the same blood group as the patient but has not been cross-matched with the patient's blood. Fully grouped and cross-matched blood takes much longer to process.

All fluids and blood products should be warmed before infusion. Critically ill patients tolerate lower haemoglobin concentrations than previously thought. During resuscitation a haemoglobin concentration of between 7 and 9 g/dl (normal range approximately 12–16 g/dl) is likely to be adequate, with the possible exception of those patients with acute myocardial infarction and unstable angina (Hebert *et al*. 1999).

If cardiac arrest occurs resuscitation should follow ALS guidelines as described in Chapter 6. Special attention should be paid to stopping blood loss and restoring the circulating volume. If cardiac arrest is associated with a penetrating chest wound an emergency thoracotomy at the scene may be life saving (Rhee *et al*. 2000). Cardiac arrest associated with trauma has a poor prognosis (Hopson *et al*. 2003).

Table 14.4 Glasgow Coma Scale.

Eyes	
Open spontaneously	4
Open to speech	3
Open to pain	2
None	1
Verbal	
Orientated	5
Confused	4
Inappropriate words	3
Incomprehensible sounds	2
None	1
Motor	
Obeys commands	6
Localises pain	5
Withdraws from pain	4
Flexion to pain	3
Extension to pain	2
None	1

D: Disability

Disability refers to the casualty's neurological status. The following need to be assessed.

- Conscious level is assessed quickly using the AVPU method (see below). The Glasgow Coma Scale (GCS) score is the preferred method for assessing conscious level (see Table 14.4). A scoring chart should be available on the resuscitation room wall. The best score is recorded. Some patients who appear deeply unconscious may respond to a painful stimulus. The lowest score that can be achieved is 3. Patients with a GCS score less than 8 are in a coma and will usually require tracheal intubation. Common causes of a low GCS score in the trauma casualty are hypovolaemia, hypoxia, head injury and drugs or alcohol.
- Pupillary reflexes – both pupils need to be assessed simultaneously. They should be equal in size. Both pupils should react when a light is shone on one eye (direct and consensual light reflex present).
- Lateralising signs – the patient should move both sides of their body.

AVPU for assessing conscious level:

A – Alert. The casualty is awake and fully orientated.
V – Vocalising. The casualty is awake and confused.
P – Pain. The casualty only responds to a painful stimulus, such as pressure on the nail bed or supra-orbital ridge.
U – Unresponsive. There is no response to painful stimuli.

If a head injury is suspected, the casualty's ABCs need to be optimised as described above to prevent further brain damage. This requires tracheal intubation with sedation and controlled ventilation if the GCS score is 8 or less. Further care needs to be discussed with a neurosurgeon. The response will include a CT scan and possible transfer to a neurosurgical centre for further management. Hypoxia and hypotension must be avoided to improve outcome in severe head injury (Chestnut *et al.* 1993). Current national guidelines for management of head injury should be followed (Scottish Intercollegiate Guidelines Network (SIGN) 2000).

Large numbers of casualties present with minor head injuries and concussion. Departments usually have guidelines to deal with these with regards to investigations (X-rays, CT scans) and admission or discharge. Those discharged after head injuries need to be supervised by a responsible adult and advised to return to the department if symptoms (including headache, blurred vision, nausea, vomiting) worsen. A head injury advice sheet with emergency contact details should be provided. Neurological status can change over time. Assessments need to be taken and recorded at regular intervals and recorded on a 'Neurological Observation' chart.

E: Exposure and environment

The casualty must be adequately exposed to allow a full head-to-toe assessment, requiring the removal of their clothes. Specially designed cutters are available to assist in this. Patient dignity must be maintained at all times. Efforts should be made to prevent hypothermia although a mild degree of hypothermia may be beneficial in head injury patients (Bernard & Buist 2003). It is therefore important not to over warm patients. The patient's temperature should be measured regularly and controlled appropriately.

Monitoring

Monitoring of the patient is required during resuscitation. The most important monitors are the members of the resuscitation team who look, listen and interact with the patient. The use of monitoring equipment allows earlier detection and measurement of physiological variables such as pulse, heart rate and blood pressure. A monitor will not tell you that the patient is bleeding or has a tension pneumothorax. It will merely alert you to any changes in physiological variables that occur with these conditions. The minimum monitoring required for the seriously injured patient includes:

- pulse rate and oxygen saturation using a pulse oximeter;
- blood pressure using an automated cuff;
- electrocardiogram (ECG) will give you the heart rate and rhythm;
- respiratory rate;
- capnography to measure end-tidal carbon dioxide concentration in the intubated ventilated patient;
- temperature monitoring – tympanic temperature probes are most commonly used to measure temperature intermittently. An oesophageal probe is best for continuous monitoring in the intubated and ventilated patient.

The record keeper should enter these details on the trauma observation chart. For an example of a trauma chart see: www.emergency-nurse.com/tchart/.

History of events

It is important that the cause of the injury is known and the exact sequence of events gives an idea of what type of injuries to expect. The mnemonic AMPLE offers a useful way of remembering the important areas of the history.

- A – Allergies
- M – Medications
- P – Past medical history

- L – Last meal
- E – Events

It is important to ensure that all the information required is obtained before paramedics or relatives leave the emergency department. It is also vital to correctly identify the casualty and affix name bands.

Adjuncts to the primary survey
To complete the primary survey of the seriously injured casualty, the following must also be considered.

- X-rays – chest and pelvic X-rays are a mandatory part of the primary survey in the seriously injured casualty. These can be taken whilst resuscitation is ongoing. Imaging for spinal fractures can wait until the patient is stabilised as long as precautions are taken to immobilise the spine. Time should not be wasted obtaining cervical spine images if this will delay treatment for life-threatening injuries.
- Nasogastric tube insertion – if the patient has a base-of-skull fracture the nasal route should be avoided.
- Urinary catheter insertion – expert help is needed if there is a pelvic fracture or evidence of urethral injury.
- Analgesia is an important part of initial treatment. Small doses of intravenous morphine can be titrated to relieve pain. Reducing fractures also reduces pain.
- There is a high risk of pressure sores developing if an injured casualty is immobilised on a long spine board. It is therefore good practice to remove the board as early as possible (Porter & Allison 2003). This requires log rolling the patient (see below).
- Further management of the seriously injured casualty often requires the involvement of a number of specialists (e.g. orthopaedic surgeons, neurosurgeons, radiologists, intensivists). It is important to contact them early if their services are likely to be required.

Secondary survey
As soon as it is confirmed that the casualty is not going to die from an immediately life-threatening injury, the secondary

survey can commence. The secondary survey is a top-to-toe, thorough front-and-back assessment of the patient and it identifies injuries that are not immediately life threatening. In some patients this will mean that the secondary survey takes place after emergency surgery for traumatic haemorrhage.

It is important to constantly review the patient during initial resuscitation. If the patient's condition deteriorates, they should be reassessed starting at the beginning of the primary survey with airway and cervical spine.

The log roll (see Figure 14.2)
The log roll allows assessment of the casualty's back. The procedure requires four helpers to roll the patient (one at the head and three along the sides of the casualty) and one person to examine the casualty. The person at the head maintains manual in-line stabilisation of the head and neck. The spine should be kept in alignment during the roll. The three team members on the side position themselves so one member is at the chest, one at the abdomen/pelvis and one at the legs. These three team members reach across the casualty to the opposite side of their body and place their hands on the casualty in preparation to log roll. On direction from the person at the head, the command is given to roll the casualty on the 'count of three'. The casualty is rolled toward the three team members and the back is inspected in detail and all clothing, straps and debris removed. The spine is palpated and the lungs auscultated. The rectum is examined to check for perineal injuries and anal tone. This is also a good time to remove the long spine board, as it is uncomfortable to lie on and can cause pressure sore development.

When the examination is complete the process is reversed and the casualty is rolled onto their back in a controlled manner, keeping the spine aligned.

Transfer and definitive care
Definitive care of the seriously injured casualty requires transfer to an operating theatre or intensive care unit (ICU), often via the radiology department for scans. This may require transfer to another hospital. Safe transfer requires:

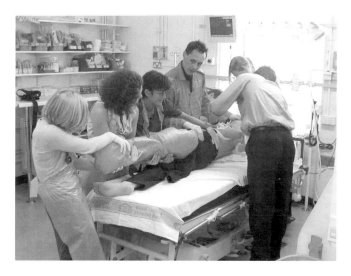

Fig. 14.2 The trauma team log rolling a casualty.

- a stable patient – this is not always possible. If a patient is hypovolaemic from a ruptured spleen rapid transfer to an operating theatre and immediate surgery is needed to stop the bleeding;
- trained personnel to monitor and manage changes in the patient's condition during transfer;
- communication – the receiving hospital or department should know that you are coming. Copies of notes, X-rays and any cross-matched blood should accompany the patient;
- monitoring equipment – the same monitoring as used in the initial management of the patient is continued during transfer. This requires robust, portable lightweight monitors with adequate battery life;
- oxygen and supplies – there should be enough oxygen in the cylinders and drug and fluid supplies to complete the journey.

Finally, the tetanus immunity status of the casualty should be checked. If there is no history available the casualty should be considered unimmunised. Antibiotic therapy needs to be started in those with wounds and injuries where there is a high risk of infection.

REVIEW OF LEARNING

❏ Trauma is a major cause of morbidity and mortality in children and young adults.

❏ Trauma care requires a multiprofessional team approach.

❏ The primary survey recognises life-threatening 'ABCD' problems.

❏ A rapid response to immediate life-threatening problems saves lives.

❏ The top-to-toe secondary survey ensures that no injuries are missed.

❏ The patient requires safe transfer for definitive care.

Case study

You are rostered to work in the emergency department resuscitation room. Ambulance control has informed the department that a casualty with multiple injuries will be arriving in approximately ten minutes. **What preparations need to be made?**

Members of the trauma team need to be alerted. The resuscitation room should always be ready to receive seriously injured patients. Team leaders should allocate tasks. Team members should don protective clothing.

A young female casualty arrives in the resuscitation room. She appears to be unconscious and looks extremely pale. She is snoring and breathing very fast. The left side of the chest is not moving. There is decreased air entry on the left side and it is hyper-resonant on percussion. Her right thigh looks swollen and deformed. The ambulance crew have already immobilised the casualty on a long spine board. She is wearing a cervical collar and her head is strapped between blocks. She is receiving oxygen.

What are the priorities in the care of the injured casualty?

A primary survey is performed using an ABCD approach. Life-threatening injuries are treated as they are identified.

- Airway with cervical spine control – the casualty is snoring. A jaw thrust is performed to avoid moving the cervical spine. The cervical spine is already immobilised using blocks and a hard collar (see Figure 14.1). High-flow oxygen is administered.
- Breathing – the patient is breathing very fast and has signs and symptoms of a left tension pneumothorax (see Table 14.2). This is treated by inserting a cannula in the left second intercostal space in the mid-clavicular line. This relives the tension pneumothorax. The circulation is assessed whilst preparing equipment to insert a chest drain on the left side.

The casualty's circulation is assessed and monitoring attached. She is very pale and has cool peripheries with a capillary refill time of three seconds. The paramedics have informed the team that her name is Penelope and that she fell off her horse. You are recording the observations: respiratory rate 30 breaths per minute, oxygen saturation 97% on 15 l/min oxygen, pulse 130 bpm, blood pressure 80/40 mmHg.

Can you explain these observations and what is the initial management?

Penelope has shock which is most likely to be due to bleeding causing hypovolaemia (see Table 14.3). The initial management includes obtaining intravenous access, sending blood for investigations, giving intravenous fluids and stopping any bleeding. There is an obvious right femoral fracture that could explain some of the blood loss.

The radiographer has taken chest and pelvic X-rays whilst resuscitation is ongoing. The chest drain has been inserted and can be seen on the chest X-ray. The pelvic X-ray shows a complex fracture which would explain the severity of the shock.

The orthopaedic surgeons stabilise the pelvic and femoral fractures in the resuscitation room as this will hopefully stop bleeding. The pelvic fracture is stabilised by applying an external fixator and the femoral fracture using a traction splint. Intravenous fluids (2000 ml warmed Hartmann's) are

Continued

given to correct the circulating volume and Penelope's observations are now: pulse 110 bpm, blood pressure 90/50. Penelope also now seems to be moaning. You have been asked to assess and monitor her neurological status. **What observations will you make?**

You need to assess her neurological status using the Glasgow Coma Scale score. It is important to check she is moving all four limbs and that her pupils are normal.

Penelope may have a spinal injury and her back needs to be examined. **How are we going to achieve this without further harming her and injuring ourselves?**

We need to log roll Penelope to assess her spine. We first explain to Penelope what we are going to do. The technique used for the log roll is described above and in Figure 14.2.

Once Penelope has been stabilised in the resuscitation room she is transferred to the radiology department for further imaging studies. She is then taken to the high dependency unit. Later that evening she has successful surgery to fix her fractures. She spends four days on the high dependency unit and a further five weeks in hospital recovering from her injuries. Six months later she is still having physiotherapy. She has missed her final term at university and is not working. Her accident has had a long-term impact on her social, psychological and physical well-being.

CONCLUSION

The initial response to resuscitating the seriously injured casualty requires prior preparation and a team approach. Early effective management may prevent death in those seriously injured patients who survive to reach hospital.

REFERENCES

American College of Surgeons (1997) *Advanced Trauma Life Support Manual*. American College of Surgeons, Chicago.

Bernard, S.A. & Buist, M. (2003) Induced hypothermia in critical care medicine: a review. *Critical Care Medicine* **31** (7), 2041–51.

Chestnut, R.M., Marshall, L.F., Klauber, M.R. *et al.* (1993) The role of secondary brain injury in determining outcome from severe head injury. *Journal of Trauma* **34** (2), 216–22.

Clancy, M. & Nolan, J. (2002) Airway management in the emergency department. *Emergency Medical Journal* **19** (1), 2–3.

Gwinnutt, C. & Driscoll, P. (2003) *Trauma Resuscitation. The Team Approach*, 2nd edn. Bios, Oxford.

Hebert, P.C., Wells, G., Blajchman, M.A. *et al.* (1999) A multicenter, randomized, controlled clinical trial of transfusion requirements in critical care. Transfusion Requirements in Critical Care Investigators, Canadian Critical Care Trials Group. *New England Journal of Medicine* **340** (6), 409–17.

Hopson, L.R., Hirsh, E., Delgado, J. *et al.*, National Association of EMS Physicians, American College of Surgeons Committee on Trauma (2003) Guidelines for withholding or termination of resuscitation in prehospital traumatic cardiopulmonary arrest: joint position statement of the National Association of EMS Physicians and the American College of Surgeons Committee on Trauma. *Journal of the American College of Surgeons* **196** (1), 106–12.

Nolan, J. (2001) Fluid resuscitation for the trauma patient. *Resuscitation* **48** (1), 57–69.

Porter, K.M. & Allison, K.P. (2003) The UK emergency department practice for spinal board unloading. Is there conformity? *Resuscitation* **58** (1), 117–20.

Revell, M., Greaves, I. & Porter, K. (2003) Endpoints for fluid resuscitation in hemorrhagic shock. *Trauma* **54** (5 suppl), S63–7.

Rhee, P.M., Acosta, J., Bridgeman, A., Wang, D., Jordan, M. & Rich, N. (2000) Survival after emergency department thoracotomy: review of published data from the past 25 years. *Journal of the American College of Surgeons* **190** (3), 288–98.

Scottish Intercollegiate Guidelines Network (SIGN) (2000) Early management of patients with head injury. Available online at: www.sign.ac.uk/guidelines/fulltext/46/index.html.

15 | Out-of-Hospital Resuscitation

INTRODUCTION

Since ancient times attempts have been made to revive casualties collapsing in the community and for centuries investigators have striven to find the most effective treatments. In the last 100 years the rise in heart disease in the industrialised nations has led to it becoming the commonest cause of cardiac arrest in the pre-hospital setting. This chapter sets out the background to current guidelines and explains the evidence that has led to their adoption. It particularly considers pre-hospital defibrillation as the single most important aspect of community resuscitation. Finally, there is discussion on developments that may improve survival in the future.

AIMS

This chapter discusses how out-of-hospital resuscitation has changed in line with the nature of sudden death.

LEARNING OUTCOMES

At the end of the chapter the learner should be able to:

❏ identify *causes* of out-of-hospital cardiac arrests;
❏ describe *factors that influence survival*;
❏ discuss *out-of-hospital basic and advanced life support*;
❏ identify why out-of-hospital resuscitation sometimes *fails to happen*;
❏ outline the development of *out-of-hospital defibrillation* and *community-based defibrillators*;
❏ discuss whether out-of-hospital resuscitation is *worthwhile*;
❏ discuss possible *developments in the future*.

OUT-OF-HOSPITAL ARRESTS

Cardiac disease accounts for more than 50% of out-of-hospital cardiac arrests and death is usually caused by a lethal tachyarrhythmia, which in turn is usually precipitated by anterior myocardial infarction (AMI) (Rosen *et al.* 2001). Tachyarrhythmias are fast unstable heart rhythms which may also be caused by electrolyte imbalance, drug toxicity and cardiomyopathies though these are much less common (Engdahl *et al.* 2002).

The true incidence of cardiac arrests presenting with ventricular fibrillation (VF) is unknown; however, a great deal of data suggest it is over 80% (Norris 1998). It is also known that the chances of successfully defibrillating the patient fall by between 7% and 10% per minute if defibrillation is delayed (Resuscitation Council UK 2000).

Survival is greater amongst patients who suffer their arrest in public places rather than at home, which is where such events more commonly occur. In one UK study 80% of instances of advanced life support (ALS) provided by paramedics were in the casualty's home (Dowie *et al.* 2003).

Predictors of likely survival of cardiac arrest (Engdahl *et al.* 2002)

Short-term survival
- Witnessed arrest
- Bystander CPR performed
- VF first recorded rhythm

Long-term survival
- Arrest caused by AMI
- Patient of moderate age
- Good heart function post event

OUT-OF-HOSPITAL BASIC LIFE SUPPORT (BLS)

Research since the 1960s has consistently confirmed that CPR is a vital holding manoeuvre to perfuse the heart and brain with oxygen, though it rarely itself restores circulation. At the time of CPR introduction to the community setting, out-of-hospital defibrillation was not developed, so the benefit of this holding manoeuvre would have been limited.

More recent research has confirmed that CPR plays another important role in prolonging the period of VF before deterioration into asystole (Holmberg *et al.* 2000). In one study shockable rhythms were present in 48% of witnessed out-of-hospital arrests where bystander CPR was being performed and in only 27% of cases where it was not (Dowie *et al.* 2003).

As discussed in the Chain of Survival (see Chapter 4), the question has arisen as to whether the lone rescuer should phone first or commence CPR. The evidence supports the recommendation for the lone rescuer to phone first prior to starting CPR. All healthcare professionals should be competent in performing CPR and should understand the rationale for seeking help first.

Dilemmas in out-of-hospital resuscitation

Despite advances in training and wider public awareness, members of the public fail to initiate CPR for many reasons.

Lack of training

The bystander may fail to initiate resuscitation due to:

- no previous training
- fear of making things worse
- panic
- fear that they may perform CPR inadequately.

Those communities where a high proportion of the population are trained to perform CPR have demonstrated higher survival rates (Eisenberg *et al.* 1990). Training will reduce the rescuer's fear of making things worse and also bolster their confidence to respond appropriately.

Reluctance to perform mouth-to-mouth ventilation

Despite the fact that the risks of infection are low (Resuscitation Council UK 2000) many people who attend CPR training express a reluctance to perform mouth-to-mouth ventilation, particularly on strangers.

In the situation where the rescuer is reluctant to perform mouth-to-mouth ventilation, chest compressions alone offer significant improvement over nothing at all. The benefit to the casualty will be further enhanced if the airway can be opened to allow the compressions to generate some tidal volume. Compression-only CPR is also used when emergency medical dispatchers provide instruction to untrained rescuers performing CPR for the first time (Resuscitation Council UK 2000).

At least one study has shown similar survival between those receiving full CPR and those receiving just chest compressions (Hallstrom *et al.* 2000).

OUT-OF-HOSPITAL ADVANCED LIFE SUPPORT (ALS)
Early defibrillation offers enormous benefit to the casualty of out-of-hospital arrest for two reasons. Firstly, it is known that these patients are in a shockable rhythm most of the time. Secondly, it is this group of pre-hospital arrest patients who are most likely to survive (Cummins *et al.* 1985). The development of defibrillator technology has allowed progress to be made in reducing the time to first shock in the out-of-hospital setting.

Nowadays it is entirely possible that the casualty in the community will receive rapid defibrillation but this has certainly not always been the case.

There have been three phases of the development of pre-hospital defibrillation:

- take the casualty to the defibrillator at the hospital;
- take the defibrillator from the hospital to the casualty;
- make defibrillators available in the community.

Taking the casualty to the defibrillator
Until pioneering work in Belfast (Pantridge & Geddes 1967), the only place a defibrillator would be found was in a hospital. It is not difficult to see that sending out an ambulance, collecting a casualty and then taking them to hospital for defibrillation was unlikely to succeed very often. Regardless of how proficient CPR had been in the intervening period, delaying advanced interventions reduced survival because:

- simple CPR (without oxygen, drugs or airway management devices) can only stave off hypoxic brain damage for a limited time;

- it will not offer any protection of the airway so it is likely that stomach contents will be aspirated into the lungs;
- CPR will delay the process of VF fading away to asystole but will not prevent it.

Taking the defibrillator to the casualty

Sudden cardiac death frequently happens to those with no previous history of heart disease and two-thirds of deaths from coronary artery disease occur in the community (Engdahl *et al.* 2002). If an AMI patient suffers a cardiac arrest in the presence of a paramedic they have a 40% or greater chance of survival to discharge (Norris 1998).

Training out-of-hospital personnel in the necessary skills of rhythm recognition and defibrillation has continued in many countries to allow them to perform unsupervised defibrillation. This has become standard practice to such an extent that it is difficult to believe that it was not always viewed this way.

Defibrillators in the community

The National Service Framework for Coronary Heart Disease states that:

> *People with suspected heart attack should receive help from an individual equipped with and appropriately trained in the use of a defibrillator within 8 minutes of calling for help, to maximise the benefits of resuscitation should it be necessary.* (DoH 2000)

A number of creative strategies have been considered in order to achieve the targets set above.

- British general practitioners – in one study, when GPs reached the scene with a defibrillator within four minutes, 90% of patients were in a shockable rhythm and 70% survived to hospital; 60% of those patients were discharged alive. One in 20 MI patients attended by a GP arrests in the doctor's presence (DoH 1999).
- Casino security guards – security guards at Las Vegas casinos were given training in the use of automated external

defibrillators (AEDs). When the first shock was delivered in under three minutes, the survival rate to discharge was 74% (Valenzuela *et al.* 2000).

- Untrained bystander defibrillation – three airports in Chicago put defibrillators in public places. Over a period of two years, 21 casualties were treated; 18 were in VF. Of these 18, ten were free of neurological impairment 12 months after the arrest. Six of the survivors were successfully defibrillated by persons with neither training nor experience of using an AED (Caffrey 2002).

First Responder schemes

First Responder schemes are joint initiatives between the ambulance service and voluntary members of the public who are provided with resuscitation training and equipment. They are called at the time the ambulance controller puts out the 999 call and may reach the casualty first, speeding up time to the delivery of the first shock.

Public access defibrillation

As stated earlier in the chapter, most arrests happen in the casualty's own home, which has led some authors to suggest putting defibrillators in the homes of at-risk individuals who could be defibrillated by their family members (Eisenberg 2001).

IS OUT-OF-HOSPITAL RESUSCITATION WORTHWHILE?

Some investigators have looked at the quality of life experienced by those who survive a cardiac arrest in the community. It is impossible for rescuers to make predictions of outcome whilst carrying out resuscitation; there is too little time and often no medical history. In terms purely of outcome, those who survive to hospital discharge have an 88% chance of living for one year and a 75% chance of five-year survival (Kuilman *et al.* 1999).

For some casualties, being left with long-term damage may be a worse outcome than dying. What is deemed an acceptable quality of life will vary between individuals. Some may feel that any sort of disability means that their life is not worth living, whereas others may accept that even profound disabilities are a price worth paying for still being alive.

One investigator who looked at how survivors viewed their own quality of life studied 50 survivors from out-of-hospital arrest and compared their quality of life against a control group. There were reduced scores for physical mobility and energy levels amongst the survivors group but factors such as anxiety, depression and general well-being were the same. Perhaps the most important statistic was that 49 out of 50 arrest survivors felt that their lives were 'worth living' (Saner *et al.* 2002).

In a small-scale study where very rapid defibrillation and impressive survival were achieved, all the survivors left hospital able to care for themselves, suggesting they had minimal neurological dysfunction (Valenzuela *et al.* 2000).

DEVELOPMENTS FOR THE FUTURE
Challenges to improving survival from cardiac arrest in the community include the following.

Training
Cities such as Seattle, where a high proportion of the public have received training in CPR, show the impact this can make on survival (Cummins *et al.* 1991). The challenge for future programmes is to train significantly more people whilst encouraging those who have previously been trained to return for annual updates. Other ways to deliver training are being explored, including replacing the instructor with a video. This system of group self-instruction has, in some studies, shown significant improvement over instructor-led classes (Woolard 2003).

Earlier defibrillation
As increasing numbers of defibrillators arrive in the community through initiatives such as First Responder and public access defibrillation schemes, it is likely that the time taken to the first shock will lessen (Davies 2002). This is due to increasing the possibility that a First Responder will arrive more quickly than the ambulance and also that the cardiac arrest will take place near to a defibrillator.

Smarter defibrillators

As defibrillator technology develops they will become not only cheaper and smaller but also smarter. The lower cost will allow greater numbers in public places and also may begin a trend for families of high-risk patients to purchase them. Advisory defibrillators currently inform the operator when a shock is appropriate. In the future the machine may also be able to analyse the rhythm while chest compressions are ongoing, thus improving perfusion to the vital organs.

There is ongoing study into the benefits of performing CPR before defibrillation in unwitnessed arrests. This is due to the risk of defibrillation shocking the patient's heart into asystole if they have had a period without CPR. Advancements in defibrillator technology may allow the machine to look at the rhythm to predict whether the shock should be delivered immediately or after a period of CPR. The voice prompts of the machine can then advise the operator whether CPR should precede defibrillation or vice versa.

Administering drugs mid-arrest, such as thrombolysis, has been shown to improve survival in individual case studies but larger studies have yet to prove their benefit (Baubin 2001).

REVIEW OF LEARNING

❏ Cardiac disease accounts for more than 50% of out-of-hospital arrests.
❏ CPR is an important holding procedure, though lack of training and reluctance to perform mouth-to-mouth ventilation may inhibit CPR delivery.
❏ Early defibrillation offers enormous benefit to the out-of-hospital arrest casualty.

CONCLUSION

Out-of-hospital cardiac arrest is an important issue due to the prevalence of cardiovascular disease in the industrialised nations, added to the fact that one-third of those suffering an AMI will die before reaching hospital. Research has clearly demonstrated that steps such as calling for help and simple basic life support can have a huge impact on successful recovery. When early defibrillation is also achieved success rates are improved still further. As increasing numbers of defibrillators appear in out-of-hospital settings, healthcare professionals must become aware of the contribution that these simple steps can make.

REFERENCES

Baubin, M. (2001) Recombinant tissue plasminogen activator during cardiopulmonary resuscitation in 108 patients with out of hospital cardiac arrest. *Resuscitation* **50**, 71–6.

Caffrey, S.L. (2002) Public use of automated external defibrillators. *New England Journal of Medicine* **347**, 1242–7.

Cummins, R.O., Eisenberg, M.S. & Hallstrom, A.P. (1985) Survival from out-of-hospital cardiac arrest with early initiation of CPR. *Annals of Emergency Medicine* **3**, 114–18.

Cummins, R.O., Ornato, J., Theis, W. & Pepe, P. (1991) Improving Survival from Sudden Cardiac Arrest: The Chain of Survival Concept. *Circulation* **83**: 1832–47.

Davies, C.S. (2002) Defibrillators in public places: the introduction of a national scheme for public access defibrillation in England. *Resuscitation* **52**, 13–21.

Department of Health (1999) *Saving Lives: Our Healthier Nation.* Department of Health, London.

Department of Health (2000) *National Service Framework for Coronary Heart Disease.* Department of Health, London.

Dowie, R., Campbell, H., Donohoe, R. & Clarke, P. (2003) 'Event tree' analysis of out of hospital cardiac arrest data: confirming the importance of bystander CPR. *Resuscitation* **56**, 173–81.

Eisenberg, M.S. (2001) Review article – cardiac resuscitation. *New England Journal of Medicine* **344**, 1304–13.

Eisenberg, M.S., Horwood, B.T., Cummins, R.O., Reynolds-Haetle, R. & Hearne, T.R. (1990) Cardiac arrest and resuscitation: a tale of 29 cities. *Annals of Emergency Medicine* **19**, 179–86.

Engdahl, J., Holmberg, M., Karlson, B.W., Luepker, R. & Herlitz, J. (2002) The epidemiology of out-of-hospital 'sudden' cardiac arrest. *Resuscitation* **52**, 235–45.

Hallstrom, A., Cobb, L., Johnson, E. & Compass, M. (2000) CPR by chest compression alone or with mouth-to-mouth ventilation. *New England Journal of Medicine* **342**, 1546–53.

Holmberg, M., Holmberg, S. & Herlitz, J. (2000) Effect of bystander CPR in out-of-hospital cardiac arrest patients in Sweden. *Resuscitation* **47**, 59–70.

Kuilman, M., Bleeker, J., Hartman, J. & Simoons, M. (1999) Long-term survival after out-of hospital cardiac arrest: an 8 year follow-up. *Resuscitation* **41**, 25–31.

Norris, R.M., on behalf of the UK Heart Attack Study Collaborative Group (1998) Fatality outside hospital from acute coronary events in three British health districts. *British Medical Journal* **316**, 1065–70.

Pantridge, J.F. & Geddes, J.S. (1967) A mobile intensive care unit in the management of myocardial infarction. *Lancet* **2** (7510): 271–3.

Resuscitation Council UK (2000) *Advanced Life Support Course Provider Manual*, 4th edn. Resuscitation Council UK, London.

Rosen, K.R., Sinz, E.H. & Castro, J. (2001) Basic and advanced life support and acute resuscitation and cardiopulmonary resuscitation. *Current Opinion in Anaesthesiology* **14**, 177–84.

Saner, H., Rodriguez, B., Kummer-Bangerter, A., Schuppel, R. & von Planta, M. (2002) Quality of life in long term survivors from out-of-hospital cardiac arrest. *Resuscitation* **53**, 7–13.

Valenzuela, T.D., Roe, D., Nichol, G., Clark, L., Spaite, D. & Hardman, R. (2000) Outcome of rapid defibrillation by security officers after cardiac arrest in casinos. *New England Journal of Medicine* **343**, 1242–7.

Woolard, M. (2003) Less teaching means more learning. *Heartstart* (British Heart Foundation), Issue 16.

Index